OXFORD MEDICAL PUBLICATIONS

Professional Education for General Practice

Professional Education for General Practice

Oxford General Practice Series • 31

PETER HAVELOCK
General Practitioner and Course Organizer, Buckinghamshire

JOHN HASLER
Regional Adviser in General Practice, Oxford

RICHARD FLEW
Associate Regional Adviser in General Practice, Oxford

DONALD McINTYRE
Reader in Educational Studies, University of Oxford

THEO SCHOFIELD
General Practitioner, Oxfordshire

JOHN TOBY
Deputy Regional Adviser in General Practice, Oxford

OXFORD   NEW YORK   TORONTO
OXFORD UNIVERSITY PRESS
1995

Oxford University Press, Great Clarendon Street, Oxford OX2 6DP

Oxford New York

Athens Auckland Bangkok Bogota Bombay
Buenos Aires Calcutta Cape Town Dar es Salaam
Delhi Florence Hong Kong stanbul Karachi
Kuala Lumpur Madras Madrid Melbourne
Mexico City Nairobi Paris Singapore
Taipei Tokyo Toronto Warsaw

and associated companies in
Berlin Ibadan

Oxford is a trade mark of Oxford University Press

Published in the United States by
Oxford University Press Inc., New York

First published 1995
Reprinted 1997

A catalogue record for this book is available from the British Library

Library of Congress Cataloging in Publication Data
Professional education for general practice / Peter Havelock . . . [et al.]
(Oxford general practice series ; no. 31)
Includes bibliographical references and index.
1. Family medicine—Study and teaching—Great Britain.
I. Havelock, Peter. II. Series.
R745.P76 1995   610'.71'141—dc20   94–42626
ISBN 0 19 262607 8

Printed in Great Britain by
Redwood Books Ltd,
Trowbridge, Wilts

Preface

General practice vocational training in the United Kingdom is a story of innovation and success. In the space of two decades, the present pattern was designed, with pilot projects in Inverness and Wessex, followed by rapid expansion of three-year schemes through the country. A varied and extensive collection of papers and books has contributed greatly to our understanding of the discipline and our ability to teach it.

But towards the end of the 1980s it was becoming apparent that vocational training needed reappraising. Many trainers had been appointed for a considerable number of years: some of them seemed to be running out of ideas. A number of them said that once the trainee had been in the practice for a few months there was a tendency for the teaching to become repetitive and stale.

We had access to trainee reports completed at the end of their training, which contained comments implying that more structure and assessments were desired.

It seemed that a course was needed for experienced trainers whose requirements were beyond the basic ones of setting up a training practice, and who might benefit from a fresh look in more detail at the educational aspects of training. So a group of us from Oxford (five from academic general practice and one from education) devised such a course, which has been running annually at Cumberland Lodge in Windsor Great Park. In it we have attempted to address what seemed to be the most pertinent issues—how to devise a curriculum and assess the learner, how to broaden the range of techniques we use, and how to enhance the quality of the training practice and of one-to-one teaching. We also looked in some detail at the ways in which adults learn, or, more particularly, at the special factors that influence how effective that learning is.

As we developed the ideas further, it seemed reasonable that we should gather them together and set them down. In the process we had to argue through the concepts in detail and make sure they were logical and useful. We were mindful, also, that ideas which might seem obvious to those of us who had explored them for many months, could be obscure and full of jargon to others. Therefore we have tried, with examples and explanations, to make this book as understandable and readable as possible, but are only too conscious of our limited success.

There are grounds for deprecating the words 'trainer' and 'trainee', with their implication of a mechanistic approach lacking imagination and an emphasis on exploration. They are terms in common parlance, however, and will be used throughout this book. More constructive alternative descriptions will be considered later (see Part 3).

The book is divided into three parts. In the first we set out the background. We look at the history of vocational training. Then we examine facets of how adult learning is influenced (and often compromised) by the fact that the learners are adult. Finally, we set out a task list for one-to-one teaching, based on arguments rooted in education.

In Part 2 we tackle the details of the various aspects of teaching and learning. We start with curriculum design and assessment and then continue with teaching methods, relationships, hospital posts, and evaluation. In Part 3 we look to the future. From an analysis of the core attributes of general practice we argue that changes are needed both now and in the longer term. The book, then, is not just about the technicalities of teaching and learning, but also an assertion that changes are needed.

Although the book is primarily directed at GP teachers, course organizers, and advisers, we hope that others will also find it useful. Trainees should be helped to realize the potential of their attachments. Many of the messages apply equally well in the hospital setting. Nor do the themes relate only to the British scene: teachers from other countries will find much to interest them.

Many people have helped us in the gestation period and it would be impossible to mention them all. Two, however, stand out. Kelly Skeff, from Stanford University, spent time with us deepening our understanding of educational method: Paul Arntson, from North Western University, Illinois, joined us for a sabbatical year and researched aspects of trainer and trainee relationships. But our special thanks are due to all those doctors who came to Cumberland Lodge, stimulated us with ideas, pointed out our failings, and gave us support for what we were doing. This book is for them and all others involved in the training of future general practitioners, whether as learners or teachers.

Oxford   P.B.H.
January 1995   J.C.H.
                                                                                                        R.F.
                                                                                                        D. McI.
                                                                                                        T.P.C.S.
                                                                                                        J.P.T.

Contents

Part 1

1 A legacy of opportunities

Before we start to consider the ways that general practice teaching should develop in the future, we must first acknowledge the substantial achievements and strengths of our present system of training. Then we need to identify those areas in which improvement is still required.

THE EVOLUTION OF GENERAL PRACTICE AND PRIMARY CARE

The start of the National Health Service (NHS) in the United Kingdom left many general practitioners confused and somewhat demoralized. Removed from the hospital service at a time when investment in specialist care was seen as a clear priority, many doctors wondered whether general practice would survive. Because of the payment system and the lack of access to diagnostic services, there was no incentive to develop new buildings or teams, or to provide a first-class clinical service.

In 1966, the new contract for general practice, developed in the context of increasing pressure from the profession, set in train developments that were to continue for the rest of the century. It made realistic for the first time the introduction of a significant number of nurses and administrative staff, and it enabled first-class buildings to be erected. It began to stimulate an interest in prevention, with the introduction of item-of-service fees for immunization and cervical cytology. Later, family planning was to become an official part of the GP contract too.

As general practice entered the eighties it was clear that to provide effective care, primary-care teams needed to adopt an active approach to their registered populations. A series of Royal College of General Practitioners (RCGP) reports (RCGP 1981–82) stimulated a much more active approach to prevention. By the end of the decade this had been developed further into secondary and tertiary prevention, with nurses increasingly supervising the follow-up of common chronic diseases. The introduction of the 1990 GP contract nudged these developments further still, with the stimulation of health promotion and disease-management clinics. Whatever the rights or wrongs of these requirements, they caused a further significant rise in the number of practice nurses. They also stimulated a large increase in practice computing. Never was it more important for doctors to be able to handle change and understand the implications of new technology.

During the 1980s the concept of primary health care was being developed. These ways in which general practice could evolve to accomodate this new thinking were described by Julian Tudor Hart in *A new kind of doctor* (1988). The essence was health professionals working as teams, based in the community, assessing the needs and capacities of their population, and developing a new partnership to work together to meet those needs. This required new skills and approaches from doctors trained in traditional clinical medicine.

It can never be certain how far these and other developments merely influenced the progress of vocational training, or how far the latter, with its framework of trainers, course organizers, and regional advisers, stimulated the thinking in general practice and formed the base from which much flowed.

THE DEVELOPMENT OF GENERAL PRACTICE AS AN ACADEMIC DISCIPLINE

Probably the most significant milestone was the formation of the College of General Practitioners in the early 1950s, which, together with its journal, began to make a major contribution to the development of a scientific approach to primary medical care.

Another major influence on general practice thinking in the 1960s was the work of Balint (1964). Working with groups of general practitioners, Michael Balint enabled them to understand their own feelings about their patients and the way in which these could be used in a positive way to influence the outcome of consultations.

One of the earliest activities needed was to map out the content of general practice in the form of incidence and prevalence of disease. Fry (1979) and Hodgkin (1985) provided statistics which are still referenced widely today and enable doctors to understand the patterns of illness seen in the community.

To understand the basis for general practice and, equally important, to be able to explain it to others, something more was needed. McWhinney (1966) was one of the earliest contributors and subsequently went on to become a powerful force in the development of family medicine in Canada. He argued that disease could not be seen on its own but was influenced by other factors to do with the patient and his surroundings. In 1972 *The future general practitioner* was published by the Royal College of General Practitioners (RCGP) copies of which are still in demand today. A working party of the RCGP divided the content of vocational training into five areas:

• Health and disease;
• human development;
• human behaviour;
• medicine and society;
• the practice.

Also included was an introduction to educational theory. This gave an important impetus to those who were designing the early vocational training programmes. Two years later another publication from the Second European Conference on the Teaching of General Practice (1974), defined the general practitioners' role and listed 21 broad aims for the teaching of new general practitioners. Pereira Gray adapted these aims to develop a system of training at Exeter (1979). This, too, addressed not only the content of general practice but educational theory, thereby underlining the need for a professional approach to learning and teaching.

THE DEVELOPMENT OF VOCATIONAL TRAINING

Looking back over two remarkable decades it is hard not to be both impressed and frustrated. The introduction of vocational training across the United Kingdom was rapid and extensive: yet in some ways progress has been much slower than was anticipated at the beginning.

During the 1950s and 1960s, experimental vocational training schemes began, notably in Scotland and Wessex. By the end of the sixties it was clear that these experiments had been a success and the introduction of schemes across the country followed quickly during the early seventies. Unlike those schemes in other parts of the world, notably North America, the British system was grafted on to existing structures. The trainee attachment arrangements to an approved practice had been incorporated in the NHS from the start, although it had largely fallen into disrepute in the fifties and sixties because of the lack of clear objectives, supervision, and support. The majority of the hospital section was composed of existing junior hospital posts, some of which were allocated to the vocational training rotations.

The existing pattern of 3 years—normally 2 years in hospital and 1 year in general practice—came about partly by popular consent and partly because by limiting the general practice period to 1 year, no extra finance needed to be authorized. In any case, at the end of the sixties the potential for the general practice component had not been fully realized and a year seemed long enough. The two sections remain in stark contrast—an increasingly busy hospital section, often with little time for planned educational sessions, and a general practice section where, in theory if not always in practice, the education can take precedence over the clinical work.

A full account of the early developments has been described by Horder and Swift (1979) and subsequent progress in the seventies and eighties by Hasler (1989).

The view of many, including the RCGP, was, and still is, that this 3 year period is too short, and over 20 years ago the Royal Commission on Medical Education (1968) recommended 5 years—3 years in hospital and 2 years in practice. In comparison with the training period for specialists, general practice training stands out as being dubiously short.

TRAINERS AND THEIR PRACTICES

Trainers and training practices are the cornerstone of vocational training. The shift from an apprenticeship that was unstructured and unsupervised, to a professional system in which trainers have developed their expertise as teachers, and practices have participated in increasingly rigorous accreditation procedures, is a key achievement. Those responsible for training practices have been required to make major changes in their organization, improve their records, and provide facilities for training, including additional consulting rooms and libraries.

Trainers are required to attend courses in teaching methods before they start, and to maintain their skills thereafter. However, it is often difficult to maintain momentum without continuing support, and the average trainers' group is not always the best option. Some trainers, even experienced ones, are worried that they are inadequate for the job, although, as we shall point out later, many of their fears are ill-founded. Nevertheless, the majority find it a great privilege and stimulus, and are looking for ways in which they can inject new ideas to keep the process fresh.

However, trainers and trainees are heavily influenced by the training practice which is there primarily to provide a clinical service. Partners vary considerably in their knowledge of, and motivation towards, training, and vary widely in their support.

Given that the trainee is technically supernumerary and brings a variety of advantages to the practice, many partnerships allow the trainer a substantial amount of time for undisturbed tutorials and outside commitments. At the other extreme, it is up to the trainer to protect the situation as best he or she can. Trainees still spend most of their time seeing patients, and their experience is variable, with the majority of patients coming mainly with self-limiting acute problems and not with continuing ones (Hasler 1983). Teamwork is variable: in many practices it is excellent, in others less so and in many there is a feeling from the other team members that they could be involved more in policy decisions, audit, and teaching. Management skills and attitudes to change are also variable. Reports from Oxford Region training practice approval visits have indicated slow progress in the field of medical audit. Fewer than half of all these practices had agreed written protocols for their clinical activities by the end of the eighties, and even fewer could produce data to demonstrate how well they were doing.

These influences play an important part in the trainees' development. Regardless of what happens on day-release courses and in tutorials, it is what happens in the practice that determines whether ideas are adopted.

Furthermore, as we explain in the next chapter, the busier the practice, the more there is interference with effective learning.

MEDICAL SCHOOL EDUCATION

In spite of the growth of university departments of general practice, the influence that these departments have had on medical education is variable. The vast majority of learning still takes place in hospital, and many students do not acquire the skills or attitudes that are needed for general practice.

Increasingly, students are expected to think critically and to understand research methodology, and they often see little evidence of scientific rigour applied in the general practices to which they are attached. That, and the way in which general practice is often viewed by senior hospital teachers, leads some to believe that, scientifically, general practice is a soft option.

But the pursuit of hospital-orientated scientific goals in itself creates problems. As Metcalfe (1989) has eloquently observed, the craft of medicine centres on decision making in situations of uncertainty, and this applies as much to specialist as to general practice. He went on, 'conventional medical education underplays this fact . . . the implicit and explicit strategy of the medical school is to reduce uncertainty by retreating to the high ground of laboratory proven, reductionist, bioscience'. Metcalfe argued that this strategy is invalid because 'all doctors have to operate in uncertainty and because moving in this direction too far takes doctors away from the patient as a person: laboratory hard ground has contributed little to health problems that are of major importance to most individuals or society as a whole'.

McCormick (1979) in an earlier publication emphasized the same point, 'Medical schools, by emphasising with good reason the scientific aspects of practice, have unwittingly diminished concern for patients as people.' Although it is now true that behaviourial sciences are assuming a larger place in the curriculum, they are still dominated by the traditional major clinical ones.

McCormick also refered to research illustrating the way in which medical students' attitudes change during training (Mann 1966). 'Candidates applying to the medical school are motivated primarily by their wish to become doctors caring for patients . . . During the six year period of study a gradual change in their attitudes and motivation occurs . . . They become less motivated to function as healers, develop to some degree even a cynical attitude in this respect, and begin to think in respect of their future in terms of scientists and researchers, who appear to them to be of a higher status in society.'

Another problem facing medical students is the requirement to acquire a large quantity of factual knowledge. In contrast, and by inference, the skills of communication, teamworking, and medical audit are regarded as less important. The point to grasp is that whether or not medical schools should change some of their strategies (and some have been looking hard at this in recent years), those of us responsible for teaching trainees must bear these issues in mind.

HOSPITAL POSTS

Immediately following graduation the young doctor is launched into an intensive work experience with rapid successions of patients and little time for reflection and exploration of major issues and feelings. He or she is expected to be macho, efficient, unflappable, and unemotional. The work is often hard, the hours long, and education and support often lacking (Reeve and Bowman 1989). (It must be said in the hospitals' defence that they face major problems in resources, both human and financial, and many consultants would like to change things if they could.) It is these young doctors who arrive breathless and sometimes confused in our practices.

What effect does this 8 years' experience have? First, it tends to create a value system where clinical knowledge and practical skills have a high priority compared with self-awareness, behavioural skills, and appropriate attitudes. Newly arrived trainees, being questioned on their priorities for the practice year, tend to reply solely in terms of more experience in clinical specialties rather than in terms of developing or sharpening skills in consulting, teamworking, evaluating work, or organization.

During the 1980s, the hospitals had to face increasing difficulties, particularly in busy specialties such as obstetrics and paediatrics. While the workload increased, the junior staffing levels were frozen and financial constraints became tighter. But the ever heavier service commitment was not the only problem. Supervision was not always satisfactory and many consultants were not familiar with principles of effective education.

This presented a real dilemma for those responsible for organizing GP training. Should they only concentrate on departments where supervision and education were good, or should they continue to accept posts in which the service work was too great and the education not always enough? And if they took the latter action, should they try and change things and risk losing the posts, or let sleeping dogs lie?

By the early nineties there was general acceptance that the education and service difficulties for Senior house officers (SHOs) had to be addressed. Furthermore, regional committees had become aware that there they had responsibility to decide which specialist-approved posts were appropriate for GP training, a responsibility vested in them in the Vocational Training Act. In the Oxford Region this resulted in a planned programme of visits to all hospital departments with GP-approved posts. At the present time there are still many challenges to be met, but there is no doubt that the mood is becoming more optimistic.

TEACHING AND LEARNING IN PRACTICE

For many trainees, their training practice attachment is the first time since entering medical school that they have had a personal tutor. Furthermore, it is likely to be the first time since qualification that they have the opportunity for protected learning time. The ways in which these opportunities are used are crucial to the effectiveness of vocational training.

In 1980 the organizers of the fourth national trainee conference at Exeter carried out an ambitious survey of trainees (Ronalds *et al*.1981), the results of which were presented to the meeting. Included in the conclusions were the fact that being able to discuss difficulties in the trainee/trainer relationship was crucial, and that teaching time was the most important single factor in determining trainee satisfaction. Feedback from the conference itself confirmed that the trainer/trainee relationship was highly important, that trainers should be trained to teach and that trainees should be assessed and given feedback.

At the end of 1982 a team from Manchester reported the results of its research into the influence of trainers on trainees (Freeman *et al*.1982). The authors concluded that the trainer's clinical knowledge and problem-solving skills in patient management were major determinants in the trainee's performance at the end of their attachment. They also concluded that although the one-to-one teaching attachment had many advantages, these could be dissipated by personality clashes between trainer and trainee. Other important factors in effective teaching and learning were: time spent in tutorial planning, the extent of trainer reading, continuing medical education, standards of record keeping, and general enthusiasm.

In 1989 another national survey, conducted by Crawley and Levin (1990), demonstrated some significant improvements in training compared with the 1980 survey. These included a greater use of videos, audit, and tutorials. However, some problems continued. Nearly a quarter of trainees felt that they did not get enough teaching from their trainer. Forty-four per cent did not have regular discussion of video- or audio-recorded consultations, and over a third had not been shown any audit. General practice study release programmes during hospital posts were poorly available and rarely attended.

A continuing study of trainees' views on completing their training year in the Oxford Region shows that the educational objectives they rate highest are managing common medical and psychosocial problems, and the lowest, almost universally, introducing change and innovation. Equally, seeing patients and immediate discussion of problems assume much higher priorities than taking part in practice audit, prepared tutorials, or carrying out projects.

Trainees are also asked for unstructured comments. Most are complimentary but one criticism is common: 'We started with a well structured and agreed tutorial programme but then it rather fell apart'; 'More long-term planning of the training would be better, especially at the beginning'; 'We should have had a structured timetable of tutorials and necessary achievements to accomplish'.

The overall planning of education in the practice has to take account of other factors. All trainees attend day release and other courses and it is important that the objectives are complementary and integrated. The effect of the practice environment has been mentioned and the practice provides many resources to reinforce tutorial messages. These resources include patients, partners and other professionals, records, registers, and written material. Many trainees in our survey comment that they would have liked partners and other professionals to be involved more in their teaching.

Quite apart from overall planning problems, there are discrepancies between trainers in what they regard as learning priorities. When Oxford Region trainers were asked to rank the 21 aims of the Second European Conference in importance there was no agreement about most of them, except knowledge of clinical medicine (Tate and Pendleton 1980). It was for this reason that the Oxford Region Course Organisers and Regional Advisers published their priority objectives for vocational training (1988), in the hope that there would be more logic and less idiosyncrasy in the choice of learning objectives. A further attempt to define a curriculum was undertaken by Samuel (1990), who argued for less obsession with detailed objectives and more concentration on competence and self-awareness.

Many of the deficiencies in general practice identified by patients are not to do with lack of clinical knowledge but lack of application. Important short-comings are related to lack of such skills as communication, management, and teamworking. It is important that these are identified early on and regarded as priorities—they will be needed throughout professional life, whereas clinical facts may be transient.

In spite of all these problems, enthusiastic trainers and practices can be proud of what they have achieved so far.

ASSESSMENT

The examination for Membership of the Royal College of General Practi-tioners has been developed into a reliable and well-respected test which is taken by the majority of trainees at the end of their training. It assesses knowledge, problem solving and critical thinking skills, and attitudes, and steps are being taken to strengthen its ability to assess clinical skills. There is a dynamic relationship between the content of the examination and the content of vocational training, sometimes leading, sometimes following, because many of the panel of examiners are also involved with training.

There is, however, a fundamental difference between general practice and all other specialties. In the latter, passing an end-point assessment set by their Royal College is essential before appointment to permanent posts. In general practice, partly due to the reluctance of the profession, no such effective hurdle exists by the early 1990s. Although, in theory, certification by trainers and consultants is supposed to stop unsatisfactory doctors entering practice as principals, nearly every doctor collects the necessary Statements of Satisfactory Completion. Confusion remains about what these statements mean, and there is a considerable discrepancy between the certification rate and the Member of the Royal College of General Practitioners (MRCGP) examination pass rate (Styles 1988). Although mandatory training was introduced at the beginning of the 1980s, it remains effectively a requirement to serve time and not to demonstrate competence.

BENEFITS OF TRAINING

While there is general agreement that vocational training is a good thing, the tangible benefits are harder to quantify, since the comparative performances of trained and untrained general practitioners would have been difficult to measure in the first place. We have already referred to changes in practices that can be seen, such as the move to more prevention, the interest in more effective supervision of chronic disease, and the increasing contribution from general practice in educational meetings and in the literature.

Perhaps the best place to look for strengths and weaknesses is in the comments of others. Cartwright and Anderson (1981) published their findings of a study of general practitioners, comparing the situation then to the mid-sixties. Although now over 10 years ago, at the time of the study vocational training for general practice was widespread and the changes introduced in the GP Charter in the sixties had been in operation for over a decade. Surprisingly, the percentage of GPs who enjoyed their work very much or moderately remained unchanged at 55 per cent and 36 per cent: neither vocational training, attendance at courses, nor RCGP membership appeared to be a factor. Between the two surveys there was no change in the proportion of patients who left the consulting room with a prescription. In the mid-sixties, a quarter of GPs considered at least half their consultations to be trivial, inappropriate, or unnecessary: over a decade later there was no change; and by the end of the seventies both doctors and patients were less likely to regard it as appropriate to consult their GP about family problems.

In a much more recent study, Rashid *et al.* (1989) found that, in the examination of general practice consultations, looking at patients' and doctors' satisfaction, patient satisfaction was generally high. In contrast, the doctors were less satisfied and were far more critical of their own ability to assess and treat patients, communicate with them, or allow them to express aspects of psychological ill-health.

In 1989 the Consumers' Association carried out a national survey of a representative sample of adults, to establish what they felt about their family doctors. The most important changes people wanted to see were more time explaining and listening, free check-ups, more choice and information about specialists, more helpful receptionists, shorter waits and more convenient surgery hours, more nurses, and more home visits. It is interesting that hardly any of these are to do primarily with clinical activities, but rather with communication, organization, and access.

We would not want to suggest from these comments that the majority of doctors are not working hard or conscientiously, or that there are widespread fundamental problems in practice. The progress in the past two decades has been impressive. However, the findings do raise questions about value systems, attitudes, and skills that vocational training might have been expected to address.

CONCLUSIONS

It is the purpose of this book to address these issues in a practical way so that trainers can make their teaching more effective. More importantly, we will argue that the considerable potential of the only supernumerary period of a general practitioner's training (an opportunity denied to most specialists) has yet to be realized. But first we need to know something of the way in which adults learn.

2 Adult and professional learning

The term 'adult learning' implies that adults learn differently from children. In fact, this is not entirely true; however, the circumstances in which the two groups find themselves do differ. The many similarities between children and adults learning include some important points: People learn best when:

- they are motivated to learn;
- what they need to learn is clear;
- different methods of learning are combined (for example by seeing, listening, talking and doing).

They need to:

- assimilate new information to make sense of it;
- transform their established way of seeing the world in order to make better sense of available information about it.

In other words, teachers need to be enthusiastic, clear about what they are trying to do, and use a range of teaching methods. They need to help learners build on their previous experience.

THE SPECIAL CIRCUMSTANCES OF ADULTS

There are five important factors relating to adults that may enhance or disrupt their learning.

Adults' concepts of themselves

When children are learning at school, the main object is to help them prepare for adulthood: as they become adults, they acquire rights and responsibilities. In the process they come to see themselves as people who have a function to perform and learning becomes a much more peripheral activity. If doing and learning come into conflict, it is the former that is likely to win.

Example:
John was in the second year of his vocational training scheme, doing 6 months in paediatrics. It was a busy job and John had been qualified long enough to feel reasonably competent as a doctor (and enjoyed the status that it brought him). He was able to get by with support from his registrar and found that attending the half-day release course was rather irksome. Sitting in the seminar

room did not seem to be as important as talking to children's parents or making decisions about emergency admissions, and his attendances at the course gradually petered out.

This point is worth emphasizing. Doctors (and general practitioners are no exception) are constantly busy, making decisions and solving problems. Trainees aspire to doing the same: the opportunity to become autonomous as soon as possible is highly alluring. If they are given the opportunity to move too fast to this position, they may be grateful at the time but the potential for their learning (which will be seen as less exciting) will be correspondingly reduced.

Self-esteem

Becoming an adult not only implies that one is there to perform a function but entitles one to be treated with respect. Adults (and especially those in professions) expect a certain status in society. If the act of learning threatens that status it is likely that the learning opportunity will be bypassed.

Example:
Fiona was in the second month of her GP year and enjoyed the autonomy of being able to consult on her own and make decisions without constantly having to refer to a more senior doctor. One Tuesday morning she was faced with a child with a rash. She thought it was probably chicken pox but not wanting to appear foolish in front of the child's mother, she decided that, rather than summon her trainer, she would pretend that she was sure of the diagnosis.

Previous experience

Adults have had wider experiences than children: they have beliefs, habits, and commitments. They have established ways of thinking about things: trainees, for example, have views about different diseases, their aetiology and prognosis. They also make sense of new experiences in the light of how they sorted out previous problems.

When the adult learner becomes busy and the pressures are on them, the more likely they are to revert to previous behaviour rather than to think whether they should be proceeding differently and contemplating new ideas.

Example:
Deidre was starting to do surgeries on her own and early on was asked to see a boy of eight with recurring headaches and abdominal pain. She had previously been a neurology registrar and spent about 30 minutes doing a full CNS examination followed by ordering investigations on the basis that it might be a cerebral tumour. Later, in discussion with her trainer, it transpired that there were several reasons why stress was the likely cause, and Deidre realized she needed to modify her approach. This she initially found difficult and when under pressure in the consultation she found herself asking direct questions about symptoms rather that discussing the causes of distress.

Context and environment

Children learn in classrooms which are designed for the purpose. In contrast, the environment in which adults work is designed for action. The average office is set up with established procedures, where people work to certain goals: whatever learning occurs is usually incidental. The contrast between the two environments is to do with attitudes and ethos as well as purpose. Novices may learn to survive and cope in places purely designed for action, but the potential for personal development will be realized much more if the environment is one in which mutual learning and development is also encouraged and nurtured.

Example:
Sue was half way through her trainee year and was impressed by the way that all the team members were encouraged to improve their performance. She was never expected to come back for a surgery after her half-day release course and found that this time was precious: she needed to think through some of the new ideas. All the doctors met each week for a clinical meeting or journal club, when everyone in turn presented material. Sue was encouraged to interrupt her trainer whenever she wanted and quite often the two of them would spend half an hour in the pub after the tutorial discussing issues.

Effective teaching practices are ones where everyone, collectively and individually, is given the opportunity for personal development. If trainees are expected to work hard without a break whenever they are not at the day-release course or in their tutorials, they may get their statutory learning time but they have no space to think through new concepts, validate new ideas, experience a working environment where learning and personal development are as important as providing a service.

The learner's agenda

Children generally accept direction about what they should learn from their teachers. Adults, on the other hand, are expected to take responsibility for what, how, and when they learn. Indeed, they normally only learn what they judge to be relevant and useful, and at a time that seems appropriate. Teachers, therefore, need to know as much about the learner's agenda as possible. If they attempt to deal with issues that are perceived as of no interest or relevance, learning is not likely to occur.

This presents adult educators with a problem. They have to work with the learner's agenda but they know that the learner cannot be allowed to dictate the educational programme completely in the early stages because the novice is not aware of everything that needs to be learnt. So the teacher has first to become informed of the learner's agenda and then seek to influence and adjust it. Ultimately, of course, learners do need to take sole responsibility for their learning, so the teacher is faced also with the need to gradually hand over power, enabling and requiring learners to take control. This transfer of control should be seen by adult educators as necessary, both out of respect for adult learners and also in order that significant learning can occur. Mezirow (1981) has listed some important points for adult educators to assimilate into their teaching:

- Progressively decrease the learner's dependency on the educator.
- Help learners to use resources—especially the experience of others and how to engage others in reciprocal learning relationships.
- Assist learners to define their learning needs—both in terms of immediate awareness and of understanding the cultural and psychological assumptions influencing their perceptions of needs.
- Assist learners to assume increasing responsibility for defining their learning objectives, planning their own learning programme, and evaluating their progress.

Example:
Debbie found that after a month, her tutorials with her trainer became somewhat confusing and frustrating. She had been used to being told what she should learn and her trainer increasingly reflected her questions back to her so that instead of being told, she had to work out herself what to do. On the other hand, she had priorities on her agenda which did not seem to be given the attention she thought they deserved. Gradually she came to appreciate what was happening. While her trainer was ensuring that certain matters were being dealt with, such as emergency medicine, communication, and teamworking skills, he was slowly helping her to acquire a more dominant role in their relationship, where she became more experienced in knowing where to go for help and in defining her own needs and objectives. By the end of the year she had not only taken complete control of her learning, but conducted a worthwhile audit which gave her a clear picture of how effectively she was performing.

Effective teachers, then, are faced with a balancing act. First, they need to be aware of their own agenda and the necessity to ensure competence. Secondly, they need to establish their learner's agenda so that they can address the trainee's priorities while seeking to negotiate certain areas in the light of their own views. Thirdly, they need to enable the relationships and roles to change as time goes by, gradually yielding power without abrogating responsibility.

THE NEW PROFESSIONAL

GP trainees are not only adult learners; they are also novices becoming initiated into a profession. Three features of their learning, particularly relevant in general practice, are that it occurs:

- after the doctor has been awarded his or her main qualification;
- in order to help the doctor acquire practical, sophisticated, intellectual, and social skills involved in the work of a professional;
- through working with experienced professionals in their normal work and workplaces.

Three widely accepted characteristics of a profession are important in this context:

Competence

Professions claim the right of control over entry to their own membership: with it goes the obligation to be accountable for the competence of that membership. So, despite everything that has been said about the nature of adult learning, those responsible for educating entrants to a profession have to ensure that these entrants develop the necessary competence.

Judgement

Professions claim that their members' decisions depend on the expert judgement of individual practitioners and that they cannot be made on the basis of standardized rules. Thus learning to be a professional includes the development of powers of judgement. It follows that training methods such as apprenticeship, when the novice learns to do things in the same way as the teacher to whom he or she is attached, are inadequate: professional learners need to discover how to excercise expert professional judgement for themselves.

Nature of the work

Professional learning, and how it can most effectively be undertaken, depends mainly on two things—knowledge and expertise. It is on these, therefore, that teachers need to focus attention.

The conventional view is that the expertise needed for a profession is based first on a well-established body of theoretical knowledge, which is then applied to specific problems. Schein (1973), for example, distinguishes three components of professional expertise:

- an underlying discipline (or basic science) component upon which practice rests;
- an applied science (or 'engineering') component from which many of the day-to-day diagnostic procedures and problem solutions are derived;
- a skills and attitudes component that concerns the actual delivery of services to the client.

The theory, in other words, is that researchers provide the basic and applied science from which solutions to the problems of practice are derived: practitioners then use their judgement in applying these solutions appropriately to specific cases. It is a view reflected in the traditional structure of medical education with its three stages of preclinical and clinical undergraduate studies, followed by training in service posts.

This approach has been seriously questioned in recent years, however, not least by Schon in his book *The reflective practitioner* (Schon 1983). Schon argues that professionals increasingly realize that they do not solve clearly understood problems much of the time but instead are confronted frequently by puzzling situations where the nature of what is going on may not be clear. General practitioners, perhaps more than any other branch of the medical profession, will recognize this scenario. They are often required to explore the interactions of economic, legal, ethical, or psychological considerations with those of physical health. The increasing difficulty of knowing what 'health' means makes the definition of problems far from straightforward. Furthermore, 'Even when a problem has been constructed it may escape the categories of applied science because it presents itself as unique or unstable . . . a physician cannot apply standard techniques to a case that is not in the books' (Schon 1983).

In practice, professionals develop expertise to deal with complex and ambiguous situations. They do so in ways that they often describe as 'professional good sense', 'intuition', and, above all, 'using one's experience'. This expertise may be referred to as *craft knowledge* (A. Tom 1984; Brown and McIntyre 1993). Much of the professionals' work seems to depend heavily on knowledge and ways of thinking which are more subtle and less dependent on academic learning than the established model of professional education would lead one to believe. This may be why practitioners (including GPs) are frequently dismissive of approaches that they perceive to be academic (K. Zeichner *et al.* 1987)

If this is the case, it becomes crucial that professionals, such as general practitioners, who work in this way and who are involved in teaching others are able to describe the nature of their expertise. One of the most characteristic features of this expertise is the fluency with which experienced practitioners tend to operate, even when the thinking required is highly complex. This fluency may hide the complexity from observers and often from the practitioners themselves. In the normal course of events there is little need for an explicit analysis of either the problem or solution; the practitioner's intuitive understanding leads him or her to an appropriate course of action. The problem for an observer or trainee is that the process may be mistakenly perceived as simple whereas it may be anything but.

This fluency is facilitated by several features of professional practice which have been consistently identified (Schon 1983; Benner 1984; Berliner 1987):

- Information gathering is highly selective.
- Uncertainty is minimized by knowing when to deal with immediate problems and when to take the long view.
- Account is taken of different contexts and of the background to the problem presented.

Experienced practitioners seem to store their knowledge in terms of images or schemes through which they recognize situations as of a particular type with appropriate needs. However unique the situation on the surface each can usually be related to others experienced previously and requiring similar action. At the very least, the previous experience acts as a starting point for choosing a solution to the problem under consideration.

What this means for professional practitioners such as general practitioners is that the development of their expertise clearly depends on their personal experience. It is known that people vary greatly in how efficient and how effective they are in learning from their experience. So a professional educational programme may perhaps best be judged by how well it enables people to do this.

FROM NOVICE TO EXPERT

However good the educational programme, novices cannot acquire professional expertise rapidly. Dreyfus and Dreyfus (1984) have developed a five-stage model of the typical process of moving from novice to expert. This model has been summarized succinctly by Benner (1984) who has herself applied it impressively (and very influentially) to nursing.

[The learner] passes through five levels of proficiency: novice, advanced beginner, competent, proficient and expert. These different levels reflect changes in three general aspects of skilled performance. One is movement from reliance on abstract principles to the use of post concrete experience as paradigms. The second is a change in the learner's perception of the demand situation, in which the situation is seen less and less as a compilation of equally relevant bits and more and more as a complete whole in which only certain parts are relevant. The third is a passage from detached observer to involved performer. The performer no longer stands outside the situation but is now engaged in the situation.

This transition that new professionals, such as trainee GPs, must go through creates a number of recurrent problems in professional learning, of which five seem to be especially important.

Taking expertise for granted

Reference has already been made to the phenomenon of experienced professionals being fluent and dealing intuitively with situations: often failing to appreciate the detail of their own problem-solving skills, they tend to refer to much of their work as 'obvious'. They may neither acquire the habit of, nor see the need for, making explicit the complexity or subtlety of what is going on. As a result, novices are often misled by the apparent simplicity of what they observe. (Indeed, the more self-critical of them tend to be puzzled at their own failure to do the same things with equal competence.) So long as the underlying complexity of professional practice goes unrecognized and unrevealed, novices not only lose the opportunity from learning from the rich, specific, and contextualized knowledge of experts, but also have difficulties in understanding the general nature of the expertise they need.

Example:
Margaret had recently been appointed as a trainer and encouraged Tom, her first trainee, to sit in with her. One day a lady patient attended who was well known to the practice with menorrhagia, depression, and diabetes, and who lived in a council house with six children. In the discussion afterwards, Margaret had to think hard so that she could explain to Tom how she had weighed up the priorities for her medical care, how these related to her social situation, how she had decided which member of the nursing team to involve, how she had formulated a plan for helping her, and how she felt about the patient as a person.

This illustrates one of the challenges facing GP trainers. It would have been easy merely to discuss the immediate problem and its solution without going through the detail of the decision-making which included important background information of which the trainee would have been unaware.

Wanting to run before walking

Novices want to be accepted and recognized as proper professionals. If they mistakenly perceive things as being relatively straightforward they want to set about their own practice in a similar way. Unfortunately, lacking the necessary experience, they may get into trouble without always realizing it. They need to recognize that, unlike experienced practitioners, they have to depend at the beginning on abstract general principles and on explicit analyses of cases. (For GP trainees this problem may be compounded by the acquisition of clinical experience in the hospital setting, some of which is inappropriate for general practice but which may encourage them to believe they are more competent than they really are.) Novices have to recognize that there is a progression to expert that includes the necessary and distinct step of being a competent novice.

Example:
Linda had been a hospital registrar prior to becoming a GP trainee. After sitting in with Malcolm, her trainer, for three consulting sessions, she was anxious to get started. The problems all seemed relatively straightforward and soon she said she was happy to see eight patients an hour. Malcolm was concerned that she seemed to be overconfident and so they both looked at a number of video consultations. It gradually dawned on Linda that she was often taking physical symptoms at face value without considering psychological and social factors: her consulting rate was then slowed down to enable her to think these issues through more carefully.

Relying on recipes

A different problem arises where a novice (or worse, a novice's teacher) believes that professional expertise can be understood as the application of a set of rules, without the use of individual professional judgement that takes account of the difference between one situation and another. Although an experienced professional does not practise properly in such a way, there are some who are ready to advise novices in terms of ready hints and tips. Novices, keen to be seen to be coping, may find security in following recipes. Indeed at this early stage, so long as the recipes are sensible they can be very helpful. If the novice assumes that this is all that is needed, however, it will prevent him or her from behaving as a learner.

It is important to realize that extensive repertoires rather than single recipes are needed. Any recipe, however sensible, has limits to the range of concerns it can provide for and the confidence that one can place in it. Someone moving from the novice stage has to become aware of the limitations of the general rules upon which he or she has initially relied.

Example:
Justin was a keen trainee and at his trainer's suggestion had worked through a logical approach to managing tonsillitis. He knew the statistical likelihood of whether it would be viral or bacterial, and decided that there was no justification for giving antibiotics in the first instance. As he became more experienced he found that applying this rule did not always work. Some mothers had other agendas, such as whether exams were looming for their children or whether the family were going abroad the next day, and gradually Justin came to use what had originally been his rule for guidance only.

Conflicting agendas

The need for learners to take responsibility for their own learning, yet for the teacher to influence it appropriately, raises questions about relationships and negotiation.

Given that the criteria and standards for competence cannot be negotiable, teachers must work out a strategy that is effective. Teachers almost universally underestimate the importance of the power differential which ensures that, even where relationships are most relaxed and friendly, their pupils remain polite and submissive about the important things. It may appear that learners have accepted what their teachers say, whereas in fact they have not. Nor can teachers try to solve this difficulty by opting out of any serious discussion about the learner's agendas and leaving it to the learners to judge for themselves what they need. Developing the learners' capacities for learner-centred education does not imply that the teachers have no input. Learners are inadequately equipped to work out everything they need in the early stages, and leaving them in charge is no way to proceed. So what can teachers do to make sure that their interventions are effective?

First, they must help learners to bring out into the open at an early stage what and how they want to learn. The difficulty should not be underestimated. Many learners (and GP trainees are no exception) have not thought through in detail what they want to learn, nor have they always worked out why they have made those choices. Still less have they considered how they learn. (These matters are referred to throughout this book as the 'learner's agenda'.)

Secondly, once teachers have established what is on their learners' agendas, they need to know in what way they should influence them. This means they must have logically derived agendas of their own, covering both content and methods of learning.

Thirdly, teachers have to find ways of bypassing the problems created by the power differential in the learner-teacher relationship. If this problem is to be solved, two things should be recognized. First, teachers and learners must be aware of the situation in general and have some understanding of how it applies to them. Secondly, it should not be left to the individual learner and teacher to find a solution on their own. Although their personal relationships and negotiation of their own plans are very important, experience suggests that an institutionalized framework is necessary. For example, one framework which has proved helpful is that of a number of stages through which it is agreed all novices should go in their learning, with different imposed requirements and increasing degrees of autonomy at successive stages.

Example:
When Melanie arrived in her training practice she was a little anxious. She had only a vague idea of what she wanted to achieve and she had heard from a friend who was half way through her trainee year in another part of the country that in that practice the trainee made all the decisions about the tutorial subjects. Her own trainer explained during the first week, however, that the local scheme trainers had agreed a staged plan for learning and assessment during the year and that in the first 3 months he would be largely determining the agenda because there were certain things he needed to know relating to her competence. Later in the year, Melanie would gradually take charge. In the meantime she found that all her queries and suggestions were met with a positive response and she soon became more confident in commenting on her trainer's thoughts.

Oversimplification

Despite its complexity (or perhaps because it is so complex that it has not been understood), professional learning has suffered from oversimplification and the reliance on one particular ('best buy') way of learning. The reality, of course, is that there is a great deal to be gained from a combination of methods. Each individual method has advantages but each also has limitations. The ways in which good practice are learned are complex and cannot usually be confined to one approach.

For example, novices who merely learn from their own experience will tend to have a fairly limited approach to problems because they are unlikely to recognize different situations or possibilities. Novices need to be helped to understand why experienced practitioners behave as they do. They can then begin to appreciate the complexities of situations and how good practice involves the need for adaptation, rich repertoires, and the recognition of various practical constraints.

However, this alone is not enough. Novices also need to test their emerging ideas against the evidence in relevant literature. If they are to develop criteria and standards for their professional work, they must be aware of the latest arguments for and against particular approaches. This means that teachers must be well informed rather than simply basing their teaching on personal experience alone.

Novices need, too, to be able to compare their experiences in detail with their peers and to use these comparisons in order to develop their understanding. For example, case discussions in day-release courses enable learners to be presented with more than one way of examining problems and to be exposed to various different attitudes. In addition to this, learners usually need to develop new practical and behavioural skills, and these will require instruction, supervision, and feedback on the part of the teacher.

So, effective learning depends among other things on:

- experience;
- reflection;
- awareness of literature;
- comparison with peers.

Effective learning also depends on a range of approaches. Four different ways of learning are described by Kolb *et al.* (1974)

- experiential—learning through activities;
- participative—involving the learner as far as possible;
- instructional—learning proceeds in stages;
- didactic—learning is based primarily on a syllabus.

Thus it is clear that a wide range of sources and methods of learning are mutually complementary and are all necessary. Two further points should be made. First, these sources and methods are not only complementary but interdependent in order to be effective. The strengths and limitations of what is learned from tapping an experienced practitioner's expertise can only be understood by submitting this learning to the kind of critical examination possible in a day-release course, and vice versa. Secondly, a wide range of sources and methods will help novices to develop the autonomous approach to learning that they will need for the rest of their careers.

Example:
Dennis attended the day-release course when they discussed epilepsy and was rather surprised when Denise, his trainer, suggested that they start the next tutorial with the same subject: he thought that it would be a waste of time to do the same thing twice. However, the tutorial started with a video of Denise dealing with a patient newly diagnosed as having epilepsy, in which she demonstrated the importance of eliciting this patient's individual concerns. Afterwards they looked through her tutorial file of articles on epilepsy, which included two highlighting areas of care to which general practitioners needed to pay particular attention. When Denise suggested that Dennis take over the care of another patient with epilepsy he began to see that it would be useful to pool all the information he had gained and see how he could make it work in practice.

CONCLUSIONS

A number of factors relating to the way adults and new professionals learn must be understood if GP trainees are to have the benefits of effective teaching and learning:

- Being a doer often conflicts with being a learner.
- Wanting to feel respected often interferes with learning.
- Hospital experience may make trainees feel inappropriately confident.
- Busy practices may interfere with learning.
- Teachers must allow learners gradually to take more control of their learning.
- Practitioners who teach must be able to dissect and describe their performance for learners.
- Learning depends on more than applying sets of rules.
- Ensuring competence and allowing novices to control their learning are both essential.
- A wide range of resources and methods must be used.
- Both the professional expertise of the individual teacher and the application of scientific knowledge are equally important.

3 Educational tasks

Vocational training for general practice is just one example of the process described in the previous chapter of adults learning a new profession. The aims of vocational training are to help trainees:

(1) acquire the abilities that enable them to perform competently the work of a general practitioner; and

(2) to be able to continue to develop and maintain that competence and to adapt to change over a professional lifetime.

This second aim requires the trainee to develop the self-awareness and attitudes that enable doctors to understand their personal involvement in practice, to overcome their limitations, and to maintain their integrity and motivation throughout a professional lifetime. These aims will be considered more fully in Chapter 4 on constructing a curriculum.

The role of the trainer is essentially to help trainees to use their training time to acquire the knowledge and skills, the critical thinking, and the personal growth that trainees will require for their professional lives. Such a broadly stated aim has the advantage of defining the limits of the trainers' responsibility and emphasizing that it is the trainee who is doing the learning and the growing, but it is of little help to the trainer in understanding how this is to be achieved.

THE EDUCATIONAL PROCESS

It is possible to use our knowledge of the stages in the educational process and our understanding of the ways in which adults learn (described in Chapter 2) to derive a series of tasks for the teacher. These can be considered both in the context of any individual teaching session or tutorial and for the whole of the training attachment.

In Chapter 2 it was shown that trainees bring to the training not only their personal attributes but also their previous experience, their aspirations, and their learning style, and that these factors influence the learning that is going to take place.

Trainers bring their personal attributes, experience, and teaching skills, as well as all the resources for learning that have been developed in the teaching practice. In addition, they bring their understanding of the aims of vocational training and of the core objectives that the trainee must be able to perform in order to practise competently.

The trainer and trainee then enter the educational process together. The trainee can state his or her agenda, and the trainer can assess his or her needs

Trainee brings

Personal attributes

Previous experience

Aspiration

Learning style

Trainer brings

Personal attributes

Experience and knowledge

Priority objectives

Teaching skills

Assessment and
negotiation

Teaching and learning

Individual curriculum

Independent practice

Continued learning

Fig. 3.1   The educational process.

in relation to the objectives. They can then negotiate the content and methods of teaching and learning, and choose appropriate resources from those that are available. For example, the trainee may ask for help with a patient who is a frequent attender. After discussion the trainer may form the view that the trainee has not detected that the patient is depressed. They may then agree to have a tutorial on depression, to video-record the next consultation with the patient, or agree that the trainee should discuss the patient with the nurse who also visits her and knows her well.

The next stage in the educational process is that the trainer and trainee together should consider what has been learnt and how effective the training has been. This requires a relationship that enables honest feedback by both parties.

The outcome of this process is that the trainee moves further towards competent practice and the ability to be aware of his or her own strengths and weaknesses, and the trainer continues to evaluate and improve the effectiveness of his or her teaching. This whole process is shown in Fig. 3.1.

TASKS FOR TEACHING AND LEARNING

Specifying these stages or processes in terms of tasks to be achieved rather than specific behaviours that must be performed acknowledges that different trainers may take very different approaches to the same end. For example, one trainer may help the trainee to learn about chronic disease care by conducting a tutorial based on some previous reading. Another may ask the trainee to sit in and observe the diabetic clinic, while a third may encourage the trainee to conduct a small audit project. Each approach may well be equally effective, although, as was suggested in Chapter 2, a combination of all three would be even more so.

Defining effective teaching in terms of tasks which are equally applicable to learning knowledge, skills, or attitudes also helps to draw together trainers who place differing degrees of importance on these areas. From this model it is possible to derive the tasks that need to be performed to be an effective teacher. The trainer will need to be able to:

(1)   define the priority objectives for learning;
(2)   identify the learner's agenda;
(3)   assess the learner's needs;
(4)   negotiate and agree the content and priorities for learning;
(5)   select and use appropriate learning methods and resources that develop the trainee's
    (a)   competence,
    (b)   critical thinking,
    (c)   Self-awareness;
(6)   provide an environment and example that reinforces the learning;
(7)   agree plans for future learning;
(8)   use time efficiently;
(9)   establish and maintain a relationship that enables the other tasks to be achieved;
(10)   evaluate the extent to which the above tasks have been achieved.

In this chapter we will consider how each of these tasks relates to the principles of adult learning described in Chapter 2. The second section of the book will describe how each of these tasks can be achieved in practice.

Define the priority objectives for learning

The work of a general practitioner is largely defined by the problems that patients present, and by the services that they require. There is considerable variation between patient populations, and between practices, and trainees need to be equipped to enter practices which may differ greatly from their training practice. Trainers need to be familiar with the core skills and understanding needed by all members of the profession. A number of publications describe the consensus views of groups of teachers, for example *The future general practitioner* (RCGP 1972), the *Exeter system of training* (Pereira Grey 1979), and the *Priority objectives of the Oxford Region* (Oxford Region Advisors and Course Organisers 1988). Familiarity with a set of aims and objectives will enable the trainers to have a benchmark against which they can assess the trainee's needs, to negotiate and plan the learning, and finally to accredit that the trainees have satisfactorily completed their training. Aims can be broad statements of intent, such as those at the beginning of this chapter, while objectives are more specific statements of what the learner should be able to do, under what conditions, and to what standard. For example, an aim might be that 'the trainee should be able to manage chronic diseases effectively', and an objective would be that 'the trainee should be able to use an ophthalmoscope to detect diabetic retinopathy in 90 per cent of cases where it exists'.

This task is discussed further in Chapter 4.

Identify the learner's agenda

The trainees have a number of agendas, and these will determine not only what they will learn, but also how they learn it. Unless what they really want to learn and their preconceptions, assumptions, and theories are made explicit, it is impossible to negotiate and to come to an agreement or contract about the teaching and learning, barriers to learning may exist and will be perpetuated.

The trainees' previous experience will have been almost entirely in hospital and they may or may not recognize its limitations. They will also have their own idea of what general practice consists of and the sort of doctor they hope to become. Once they have started in practice, however, their agenda is more likely to be dominated by the immediate cases and problems that they have seen and the difficulties they have encountered. It is therefore important to achieve a balance between these short- and long-term agendas.

Other important dimensions of the trainees' agenda are their preconceptions about their role as both learner and doer in the practice, and their preferred methods of learning. Their previous experience will tend to lead them to expect immediate and full responsibility for patient care, but to take a passive role in their education. However, all generalizations are dangerous, which is why it is so important to explore each individual's own agenda before proceeding to the next tasks.

This task is discussed further in Chapter 7.

Identifying the learner's needs

The degree to which the learner's own agenda is the same as the learner's actual needs depends largely on his or her self-awareness and knowledge of what is required to function as a general practitioner. In the short term, when the trainee presents with a problem case or topic, the trainer must not only listen to his or her own ideas or concerns, but also be able to assess where the real difficulties lie. This will be done in the light of the trainer's knowledge and experience of what is required to be able to handle this problem competently; in other words the objectives for training in this area, as described in the first task (p. 00).

This assessment must be as objective and reliable as possible and will depend on information obtained from a wide variety of sources. Some of this information will be collected during normal teaching, for example case discussions or viewing recorded consultations. Some may need more formal assessment tools, for example a multiple-choice paper. The essential points are that these assessments need to be explicit, recorded, shared with the trainee, and, most importantly, be related to the curriculum and contribute to its planning.

In the longer term, the trainer needs to be able to assess the progress the trainee is making towards being able to achieve these core objectives. This needs to be set against the expected progress at each stage in training and it is therefore very helpful to have a plan or curriculum that specifies this.

The three stages that the trainee moves through can be identified as:

- *The new trainee*, being assessed and introduced to the practice.
- *The practising trainee*, seeing patients, playing a full part in the activities of the practice, and learning the core knowledge, skills, and attitudes required for general practice.
- *The practitioner*, now more able to choose the direction of their learning and able to allocate time appropriately.

This is discussed further in Chapters 4 and 5.

Negotiate the content, methods, and priorities for learning

It is very easy to embark upon a teaching programme based on assumptions which are not stated and which later turn out not to be shared. The first requirement is that these assumptions should be made explicit and should cover not only the teacher's objectives, the learner's agenda, and the learner's needs, but also the order of priorities in which they should be approached, the way that time and resources are to be used, and the responsibilities of each party in the relationship.

This negotiation can apply to an individual teaching session or to the planning of the training year. During the year, however, this contract needs to be re-examined at regular intervals in the light of both the trainer's and the trainee's evaluation of progress and difficulties so far.

This mutual evaluation will help to overcome one of the difficulties in these negotiations—that the trainer starts out with greater knowledge, and certainly with greater power and control over the teaching, and yet the trainee should gradually learn to develop control over his or her learning, as emphasized in Chapter 2.

Apart from developing a mutually honest critical relationship, the trainer can also surrender power by indicating when he or she believes that the trainee has achieved a basic level of competence, and the direction of learning can then be determined by the preferences of the trainee. This change in the relationship and direction of the learning is much more likely to take place if it is specifically stated and negotiated.

This task is discussed further in Chapter 7.

Selecting and using appropriate learning methods and resources

The trainee can use a wide variety of learning methods for example seeing patients, observation and discussion in the practice, day-release courses, and independent reading. The majority of these do not depend on the active involvement of the trainer. The trainer's role is therefore more that of a coach or manager of learning, guiding trainees in their development and in the choice of activities. This process of setting the agenda and selecting appropriate methods of learning produces a planned curriculum which can guide the activities of both the trainer and trainee.

We have already argued that trainees not only need to develop competence to practice now but also the understanding and awareness required to continue to develop later on. This also places a premium on methods of active learning. Trainees will, however, have their own preferred learning style and may initially wish to be taught some things directly. Again it may be helpful at the outset to specify the different stages of learning and the expectation that as each stage of the training is completed control will shift more to the learner.

This task is discussed further in Chapters 6–9.

Provide an environment and example

The power of modelling as a method of learning has been discussed in Chapter 2. The trainer and the whole practice team provide models of attitudes and practice as well as the experience from which the trainee is learning. If the messages the trainee receives from his teaching and from the practice are the same, they reinforce each other powerfully. If, however, the teaching is not related to experience, or if the practice is providing quite a different model of care, trainees will have to make choices about what they intend to learn, and the practice will tend to dominate.

The trainee will also learn from the value that the practice places on education and time for reflection. It is particularly important that the trainer and partners do not provide a model of being too busy to think, read, or discuss their own dilemmas.

The way that trainees are accepted by other members of the practice team will also influence their attitudes and their behaviour. There is a danger that the condition of acceptance can involve making a full contribution to patient care, and unless the legitimacy of time spent learning is agreed by the whole practice, the education will be undermined.

This task is discussed further in Chapters 6 and 8.

Agree plans for future learning

Any experience, teaching session, or assessment can identify unanswered questions, strengths to be built on, and weaknesses to be corrected. Reflecting and asking the questions 'What have you learnt?' and 'What do you now need to do?' will increase the value of any learning opportunity. Agreeing plans for future activity, including any division of responsibility and resources to be used, not only enables future learning to take place, but also emphasizes the continuing nature of education.

This task is discussed further in Chapter 7.

Use time effectively

Any individual teaching session has a limit on its length, and part of the negotiation of content and priorities must include the way that this time is used, so that priority agendas are met. The way that time for education is allocated within the year as a whole and within each working week should also be negotiated.

This task is discussed further in Chapter 7.

Establishing and maintaining a relationship

There is a temptation to define a 'good' trainer/trainee relationship as one in which both parties feel warmly about the other and avoiding anything that might disrupt this. An 'effective' relationship is, however, one that enables the other tasks of teaching to be achieved. This is therefore one in which the trainee's ideas are respected and negotiation can take place; one in which the trainer can assess the trainee, and the trainee can evaluate the teacher, and both give positive feedback to each other; and one in which feelings and attitudes can be explored openly. This relationship will evolve over time, and this should allow trainees to develop from their initial introductory stage to the practising trainee stage, and then to that of the more independent practitioner. If the transition between these phases is clearly marked by an assessment and explicit negotiation, this will allow the nature of the relationship between the trainer and trainee to develop and change appropriately.

This task is discussed further in Chapter 8.

Evaluate the effectiveness of the learning and teaching

Evaluation seeks to answer the questions 'How effective is the teaching?', and 'How could it be improved?'. This can be applied to an individual session or to the whole programme, and evaluation can cover aspects of structure, for example resources in the training practice, the process of the teaching, or its outcome.

Process evaluations, in which the learners, the teacher, or an external observer comment on the content, methods, relevance, or value of the teaching are the most common form of evaluation, and can have the advantage of indicating areas or directions for change. This should be a mutual activity in which each party assesses its own and the other person's contribution to the learning. Encouraging this mutual evaluation helps to develop the open negotiation discussed above and allows the teacher to model the process of self-evaluation and the acknowledgement of weaknesses.

Evaluating teaching by assessing outcomes in the learner may appear to be more rigorous, and it can be argued that the only true evaluation of teaching is how much the learner has learnt. However, this ignores the crucial contribution of the learner and assumes that the trainer is taking responsibility for the trainee's learning. Outcome evaluations also require a design that can relate changes in the learners to the teaching they have received, but such controlled conditions are not usually feasible.

This task is discussed further in Chapter 11.

CONCLUSIONS

These 10 tasks can provide a coherent statement of what is required to be effective both in an individual teaching session and during a trainee's attachment. Subsequent chapters will consider each of these tasks in more detail and discuss the ways in which they can be achieved.

Part 2

4 Constructing a curriculum

Two aims of vocational training were identified at the beginning of Chapter 3; first, that at the end of training the trainee will have acquired the ability to perform the work of general practitioner competently, and, secondly, that the trainee will be able to continue, develop, and maintain that competence, and to adapt to change over a professional lifetime. In this chapter we shall review briefly some previous work that attempts to define a curriculum for general practice education, and suggest a three-stage model for the trainee year. Then we shall examine the content and context of general practice and the attributes needed of the doctor.

One of the difficulties in the design of vocational training has been a sense of polarization between training doctors for the job and ensuring that they can continue to train and adapt themselves later on. One is concerned particularly with content, the other with skills; one is teacher-directed, the other learner-directed. Both are needed; a concern to develop learner-directed education as opposed to teacher-directed training can create a reluctance to define the core content of the work of a general practitioner and lead to the rejection of the idea of a planned curriculum for training.

We think that this dichotomy is a false one and that it remains essential to define, and make explicit, what trainees are expected to have learnt at the end of their training. Trainers have a responsibility to trainees to help them use their time as constructively as possible, and to the public to be able to assure them that doctors entering practice are competent in the care that they are undertaking. In addition, it is possible to lose sight of those very attributes that are valued most highly, such as self-awareness, enthusiasm, and the ability to evaluate one's work in the light of new information, if they are not defined and methods of fostering them considered when teaching plans are drawn up.

Another reason why attempts to define a curriculum for general practitioner training have not been accepted widely is that it can very easily turn out to be a long check-list of topics to be covered; this can be very daunting at the outset of training and often loses some of the most important educational aims. On the other hand, without a curriculum the learning can be directed solely by the cases and problems that the trainee sees; this experience may be very skewed and important areas of learning practice can be omitted.

REVIEW OF CURRICULA

The *Future general practitioner* (RCGP 1972) started with a job description of a general practitioner and from this derived 11 goals for vocational training. These were that at the end of training the trainees should be able to demonstrate:

(1) ability to make diagnoses about their patients which are expressed simultaneously in physical, psychological, and social terms;
(2) how their recognition of the patient as a unique individual modifies the ways in which they elicit data and make hypotheses about the nature of the illness and its management;
(3) that they can make decisions about every problem that patients present to them;
(4) their understanding and use of the time scale that is peculiar to general practice;
(5) their understanding of the way that interpersonal relationships within the family can cause illness or alter its presentation, course, and management;
(6) their understanding of the relationship between health and illness on the one hand and the social characteristics of patients on the other;
(7) their knowledge and use of the wide range of interventions available to them;
(8) the knowledge and appropriate use of skills of practice management;
(9) that they recognize their continued educational needs;
(10) that they understand the basic methods of research as applied to general practice; and
(11) that they are willing and able critically to audit their own work.

It is remarkable how well these goals have stood the test of time, but interesting to note that there is little mention of care for the registered population, or of health promotion. The implication of these goals is that a curriculum must be derived from the current description of the work of a general practitioner. A similar approach was taken by the Leeuwenhorst Working Party (Second European Conference on the Teaching of General Practice 1974) who produced an agreed job description and from this derived a series of aims classified into knowledge, skills, and attitudes.

In its *System of training for general practice* (Pereira Gray 1979) the Exeter University Department of General Practice produced a selective list of its own aims. These were that the trainee should demonstrate his or her ability to:

(1) know what it feels like to be a patient;
(2) maintain the dignity of the patient in all conditions;
(3) practice patient-centred medicine;
(4) identify his or her learning needs;
(5) remedy his or her learning needs;
(6) assess himself/herself objectively after learning;
(7) analyse accurately his/her doctor–patient relationships;
(8) understand illness as deeply in terms of the patient's behaviour as in terms of the patient's pathology;
(9) assess accurately the capacity of a home/household to care for one of its sick members;

(10) offer, in more than half of an unselected series of consultations in general practice, practical preventive medical advice to patients;
(11) regard general practice as a branch of medicine in its own right with its own body of knowledge, skills, and attitudes;
(12) tolerate uncertainty;
(13) promote the patient's autonomy;
(14) read and analyse critically the literature of general practice;
(15) regard his or her list of patients as a population at risk for which the doctor is responsible, whether or not they happen to be consulting;
(16) analyse a problem in medical care, devise a research project to investigate it, gather and interpret data, interpret these, and present a report of the study.

The author points out that this list is not a comprehensive or coherent statement of the attributes of a competent trainee at the end of training, but rather describes the added value that training in the university department at Exeter would give to an already competent doctor. Many of these attributes are attitudinal, but the authors argued that the greatest difference between trainers and trainees lay in their problem-solving skills and attitudes.

The Oxford Region Course Organisers and Regional Advisors Group has published a set of priority objectives (1988) which the members claimed were valid, important, feasible, and assessable. These objectives were derived from a consideration of the needs that general practitioners had to meet, both now and in the future, and were grouped under five headings (see Appendix I):

(1) Patient care;
(2) Communication;
(3) Organization;
(4) Professional values; and
(5) Personal and professional growth.

Other major influences on what trainees learn are the examinations that they sit. The panel of examiners of the Royal College of General Practitioners has used the Oxford headings in planning the oral section of the College membership examination.

One problem, however, is that all these models include comprehensive lists of attributes which tend to be rather daunting and appear not to be as helpful as they might be. In addition, a missing dimension is the changing situation for the trainee as the year goes by.

The Royal College of Australian General Practitioners also used a three-dimensional model of general family practice, describing the dimensions as clinical competencies, intellectual skills, and health management skills (Fabb *et al.* 1976).

All these models seek to define objectives for the end point of vocational training. The common thread is the need to describe the job of established general practitioners and the problems that they will face. As the scope of general practice is continually developing, there is a need for an evolutionary process to create a dynamic curriculum that is reflected both in the training and in the end-point assessment. A recent example is the way that performance review and audit have developed from an activity of innovative practitioners, through the Royal College of General Practitioners Quality Initiative, to now being a crucial part of training, training practice assessments, and of the MRCGP examination.

In the previous chapter we defined the first task for all trainers in the provision of one-to-one learning as defining the priority objectives. In other words, regardless of the individual trainee, what is it that all trainees need to achieve by the end? This is the starting point for subsequent negotiation over individual agendas. It is tempting to believe that one particular model or list could simply be given to each trainee on appointment. But since the curriculum does evolve over time, and because individual trainers need to be involved in the process of constructing their priority objectives, we believe that each trainer should devise his or her own list. However, in so doing, trainers must ensure that their lists are balanced and take account of current thinking and the published work to which we have already referred.

A THREE-STAGE MODEL OF TRAINING

Trainees enter general practice having undertaken a number of hospital posts in which they will have acquired a range of clinical, interpersonal, and evaluative skills. The degree to which this experience has been planned to be relevant to general practice is very variable and what the individual has chosen to learn will depend on his or her own preferences. They may well have had no experience of general practice other than as an undergraduate medical student. We said in Chapter 2 that novices cannot acquire professional expertise quickly and that it has been found helpful to let them progress through stages. We suggest three stages for the trainee year.

The new trainee entering the practice will go through a stage of initial orientation and assessment when the trainer needs to establish that the trainee is able to see patients on his or her own and to handle emergencies in the context of general practice. This phase may be quite short but it is the time when relationships are formed, agendas are negotiated, and the next stage of training is planned.

The practising trainee will see patients and take a full part in the activities of the practice. Much of the learning during this phase will be determined by the patients that the trainee sees. But during the teaching trainers will also need to check that the trainee is competent in all the key areas. This may sound very prescriptive, but trainees have to learn what they will require in order to meet the needs of their patients. Equally, trainers have a responsibility to the public for assessing trainees and accrediting their satisfactory completion of training. Another advantage of defining this second phase of training clearly is that it then becomes possible to determine when it has been completed. Some trainees may not become fully competent until their training is nearly completed, but for many there is a danger that the training and the patients that they see become repetitive and the opportunities for broader development are lost.

During the third phase of training as a *practitioner* there should be more opportunity for trainees to set their own direction of development and their own agenda for learning. This, of course, has implications for the way trainees spend their time and raises questions about the educational value of repeated surgeries in which large numbers of patients with the same conditions are being seen. Trainees may in fact find it more demanding to be required to direct their own learning and manage their own time, but these are abilities that it is desirable to acquire.

Defining these stages means that everything does not need to be covered in the first tutorial, and the same topic can be revisited with different aims each time. To take diabetic care as an example, the trainer needs to check that the new trainee is able to handle diabetic emergencies. At the end of the practising trainee stage the trainee should be able to manage the organized care of diabetic patients. The trainer may have to check that the trainee is able to initiate management in a newly diagnosed patient, as the opportunity to do this may not have occurred. During the practitioner stage, the trainee may choose to take this further by auditing the work of the diabetic clinic, while another might choose to study methods of patient education and small-group teaching (see Appendices III and IV).

The transition between these stages in training should be explicitly stated and marked by a 'rite of passage' so that the relationship between the trainer and the trainee is allowed to develop appropriately. For example, during the new trainee stage the trainer may wish to be told about all the patients that the trainee sees. During the practising trainee stage it would be up to the trainee to ask for supervision or help when he or she feels it is needed. In this stage the trainer will be principally responsible for directing the learning agenda, and assessment will play an important part in this. In the practitioner stage trainees will review their own progress at achieving their own goals. Trainees may also need an explicit statement that once they have demonstrated their competence they do not need to continue to repeat this by repetitive work. This matter will be discussed more fully in the next chapter.

DEVELOPING COMPETENCE

In the three-stage model the trainer is able to define the competence required by the trainee at each stage of training. Competence can defined as the *'possession of the abilities required to manage a particular problem in a*

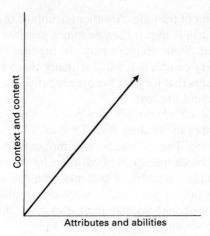

Fig. 4.1 Developing competence.

particular context. The development of competence has two dimensions, demonstrated diagrammatically in Fig. 4.1. The first is the developing range of contexts in which the practitioner will work and the content of each, and the second is the attributes and abilities required for competence in each of these areas. This framework draws upon some of the models of curricula and development which were described earlier in the chapter and will now be described in more detail.

CONTEXT AND CONTENT OF PRACTICE

The widening range of contexts or situations within which the trainee will be required to practice now and in the foreseeable future are:

- care of individual patients;
- care of groups of patients;
- the practice population;
- practice and health-care team;
- the community and profession.

The first context for a trainee is *care of individual patients* during consultations and during episodes of illness. When drawing up a curriculum it is not necessary to list every possible diagnosis that may present, because many of the skills required are used for more than one problem. On the other hand, common things are commonplace and some diagnoses have a greater significance than others. A trainer may, for example, wish to check that the trainee is capable of dealing with a selection of common emergencies before he or she goes on call, and that the trainee has developed a well-thought-through approach to the management of problems common in general practice.

There are several *groups of patients* for which general practitioners are required to deliver services over and above the demand-led care in individual consultations. These include the organized care of patients with chronic diseases, family planning, antenatal care, childhood surveillance, well-woman and well-man care, and care and surveillance of the elderly. Some groups of patients with mental health problems (for example, anxiety, depression, or bereavement) may also benefit from group rather than individual approaches to their problem.

Some of these services are covered by the new contract for general practice, but even if they are not, patients are entitled to expect a full range of services from their practice and trainers have a responsibility for ensuring that their trainees will be able to deliver these services.

Julian Tudor Hart in his important book *A new kind of doctor* (1988) argued that general practitioners also have a responsibility to their *practice population* to determine its state of health, to identify needs, and to plan services to meet these needs. This public health role has become more important with the inclusion of health promotion as a core responsibility in the new GP contract and the NHS reforms in which purchasers base their decisions on assessment of need. This requires basic epidemiological skills of population rather than personal medicine, for example as described by Morrell in his book *Epidemiology in general practice* (1988).

All general practitioners work in the context of a *practice and a team*, and the ability to provide organized care and a full range of services depends on practice management and teamwork. The pace of evolution and change is continually quickening and the ability to manage change in practice is increasingly crucial. One dimension of this is the revolution in information technology which is beginning to affect the way that general practitioners work. The skills required to implement and to use this technology will be essential in the near future, both for trainers and for trainees.

General practitioners also work in the wider context of their *community and profession*. Primary health care has the opportunity to ensure that the services it provides meet the community's needs and to involve and to empower the community itself to provide care and tackle health problems. This collaborative community-orientated health care is increasingly important as one appreciates the multifactorial causes of most health problems and the limitations of curative medicine in tackling them. At a national level, the medical profession in the United Kingdom has a credible record as an advocate on such problems as smoking, alcohol, and road safety, whereas the potential contribution of similar local initiatives is largely unrealized.

DEVELOPING ATTRIBUTES AND ABILITIES

The attributes and abilities that a trainee will need to develop include:

* knowledge;
* clinical skills;
* problem solving and decision making;
* interpersonal skills;
* management skills;
* evaluation and critical thinking;
* values and attitudes;
* personal understanding.

This list is based on Bloom's taxonomy of educational objectives (1972). This divides objectives into the areas of knowledge, skills, and attitudes, and describes the development from knowledge, through its comprehension and application, to the process of analysis, synthesis, and evaluation. The list is hierarchical to an extent; for instance, acquiring skills is dependent on first having knowledge.

The *knowledge and skills* required for clinical care may have been acquired by trainees during their hospital experience, but this is by no means certain, particularly as many problems are now managed entirely in general practice. The skills to provide some services, for example, childhood surveillance and minor operations, may also need to be acquired in training and should form part of the core curriculum.

The ability to apply knowledge and skills to *problem solving and decision making* is of a higher order than simply possessing the knowledge and skills. It is clearly essential but often difficulty to define. It includes the ability to recognize cues, to generate appropriate hypotheses, to gather information to test these hypotheses, to generate a range of options for management, and to apply criteria to the selection from these options. As we described in Chapter 2, experienced practitioners often find it difficult to describe the way they solve problems and make decisions; it is one of the attributes of an experienced trainer that he or she can explore these areas with trainees. The problem solving and decision making are often less intuitive in the context of population, care, or practice management, but again need to be explicitly discussed or learnt.

Interpersonal skills are crucial in all contexts of the work of general practitioners. While the approaches to learning and teaching consultation skills are well developed (Pendleton *et al.* 1984), trainees also need to acquire other skills such as teamwork, small-group discussion, written communication, and verbal presentation. Many opportunities exist in practice for acquiring these skills, but unless the need for them is explicitly stated these opportunities may be missed.

Effective *management* requires a particular range of skills, including the ability to manage oneself and one's time, strategic planning, and the management of change. At the present time this is the area in which many trainees report they feel most deficient at the end of their training. Throughout the development of vocational training GP teachers worked closely with other disciplines to define which of their skills were relevant. Management is clearly one area where there is scope for continued development.

The ability to *evaluate and to think critically* about one's work is important for the continued development of any professional. Much current practice deserves critical scrutiny and we anticipate that the rate of change that trainees will experience during their professional lifetimes will be even faster than it is now. Despite the increased influence of controlled clinical trials, there is still a susceptibility to uncritical enthusiasm, for example for health checks, and many deficiencies stem from a failure to apply existing knowledge rather than the lack of knowledge itself.

While recent changes in the examination for the Membership of the Royal College of General Practitioners, introducing a critical reading paper, are welcome, there is a danger that this can be seen as a separate activity rather than something that should permeate the whole of medical practice.

The whole direction of practice also depends on *values and attitudes*. One of the great strengths of the *What sort of doctor?* (RCGP 1985) approach to assessing quality of care in general practice was its explicit statements about the professional values that underpin the work of the general practitioner: doctors' perception of their roles in relation to individual patients and to the practice community; their ideals and sense of priorities; the spirit that motivates and guides the gradual evolution of their practice. These values affect work in each of the contexts that we have described. For example, doctors who see their role as very powerful and controlling may have difficulties in sharing decisions with patients, getting involved in teamwork, and empowering the community in health care.

A final dimension is the growth and maintenance of doctors as people and their *personal understanding* of the relationship between themselves and their work. Doctors as a group have a very poor record in maintaining their own physical and mental health, and many subscribe to an ethos that makes it difficult to recognize and talk about their stresses and to ask for help or support. The skills of coping with the stress of consulting and medical practice were described as 'housekeeping' in Roger Neighbour's book *The inner consultation* (1987). Again, the skill of monitoring how one reacts to other people and how others react to oneself should not be seen in isolation but as one that is required for all the contexts of practice.

PRACTICAL IMPLICATIONS

It should now be possible to take any particular topic, such as the earlier example of diabetic care, and to consider in what contexts a new trainee, a practising trainee, and a practitioner trainee at the end of his or her training may be required to operate, and then the attributes he or she will require to be effective in each of these areas.

A *new trainee* would need to be able to manage a diabetic emergency and to diagnose a patient presenting with diabetes. To do this would require some core knowledge and clinical skills.

A *practising trainee* would not only be able to manage the individual patient but also organize the long-term care of this group of patients and consider the policies for screening and case finding in the practice.

Trainees at the end of training (*practitioners*) would also need to be able to work with others to review the literature, create a protocol and evaluate the clinic, and manage the process of change in organizing and setting up such a clinic. This would require a wider range of interpersonal and management skills, and attitudes that place value on teamwork, patient involvement, and auditing care. Many of these attributes are transferable to other situations, and will be developed during the practitioner phase of training when the trainee may well have chosen to work on a single topic in greater depth.

If a trainer uses a range of worked examples in the way that has been described, then he or she will be able to create a curriculum that covers the full range of the trainee's learning needs.

CONCLUSION

Trainers should:

- construct an explicit list of priority objectives that all trainees should achieve, based on current thinking and published work;
- consider the trainee year in three stages and mark the transitions between these stages clearly;
- consider both the content and context of practice and the attributes and abilities of the doctor.

Appendices III and IV give two examples of staging.

5 Assessment for learning

Chapter 4 discussed what trainees need to learn, and a three-stage model for the trainee year was suggested. In this chapter ways of establishing the trainee's strengths and weaknesses, and how to measure his or her progress will be discussed. This process of 'assessment' must be distinguished from 'evaluation', which refers to a review of the teaching process. In other words, assessment looks at the trainee: evaluation looks at the trainer and training package—this is examined in detail in Chapter 11.

This chapter will address three principal issues. We shall examine briefly the different reasons for assessment and the difficulties facing trainers, and then spend most of the chapter looking at what is involved in constructing an assessment package. We shall stress the link between curriculum planning and assessment and list the characteristics of an effective package.

ASSESSMENT FOR DIFFERENT REASONS

Discussion of this topic requires some definitions. Assessment is concerned with two quite separate issues. The first is how to make the best educational use of training, and the usual term for this is 'formative assessment' (also known as 'educational assessment'), which is what this chapter is about. There is a second issue, however, which is whether the doctor is fit to be let loose on the public. It is the responsibility of the medical profession to ensure that patients receive good care: we have already highlighted the trainer's responsibility to ensure that trainees become competent. Deciding whether a trainee is good enough to become a principal general practitioner, i.e. whether the course has been completed satisfactorily, is generally known as 'summative assessment' although a better word might be 'accreditation'. At the time of writing, various steps are being taken to develop some kind of nationally recognized assessment which does not leave the sole responsibility with the trainer. Clearly there is some overlap between these two forms of assessment. What trainers learn about a trainee during the year will guide them in what they say in their references and in signing the declaration of satisfactory completion of training. Nevertheless, it is important to try to keep the two types of assessment separate because they are likely to produce completely opposite sorts of behaviour in a trainee.

When trainees are sitting the MRCGP (or when they think trainers may be weighing up what to say in their references), they will endeavour to conceal gaps in their knowledge or skills. However, if a good learning/teaching relationship exists in the tutorials, trainees will want to disclose deficiencies so as to get the best value from the teaching sessions.

DIFFICULTIES FOR TRAINERS

The reasons that some trainers have problems with assessment can usefully be separated into two groups, which we have called procedural and interpersonal.

Procedural

Time

Detailed assessment of a trainee takes a great deal of time, especially at the beginning. However, time spent on identifying strengths and weaknesses will pay dividends in terms of the most relevant and productive learning.

Lack of clear objectives

If detailed thought has not been given to what the trainees should achieve by the end of their course, assessment will be difficult. Statements like 'I want him to be a safe doctor able to cope with all common conditions', do not help very much. What is safe? How common is common? However, if, there are some fairly detailed targets, such as 'She must be able to audit her own work', or 'He must be able to establish patients' ideas, concerns, and expectations' (see Chapter 4), it will be clear what to look for when making assessments.

Confusion over different components

Look at this diagram, it shows the steps in assessment that people often confuse:

Clarifying objectives
Collecting information
Making decisions
Recording the results
Giving feedback
Making plans

Many assessment packages do not address all these steps individually and adequately so it is hardly surprising that trainers sometimes get muddled. Some of these steps are examined in more detail later in this chapter.

Interpersonal

Threat

Assessing peoples' performance is potentially threatening. What weaknesses will be discovered? Will one be able to cope with what is found? ('I don't think she is much good at reading, but nor am I, so let's keep out of it!'). Things may look just as bad from the trainee's point of view ('Do I really want to raise this issue with may trainer?').

Giving feedback

Part of the threat is not knowing what might be found, but, equally, many trainers have difficulty in giving feedback to trainees about their performance. Later in the chapter we will say more about this and how to make it easier.

Hierarchy and structure

Some general practitioners seem to dislike anything that smacks of hierarchy ('We are all equal here—think of yourself as a member of the partnership'; clearly, the trainee can do no such thing). This feeling that everyone is equal, that everything should be governed by consensus, and that no one should tell anyone else what to do dies hard amongst some GPs.

Professional people in many other walks of life, such as commerce and business, are used to having their performance assessed, and the need for some form of structure where these issues can be explored is readily accepted. It is helpful if trainers make it clear at the outset to trainees that although the latter are colleagues, assessment and feedback is essential if the year is to be used to its best advantage.

EDUCATIONAL ASSESSMENT

Assessment for planning education should answer important questions: where is the trainee now? Where does the trainee go next? Assessment methods include all the activities trainers undertake in-house as part of the training. The most common ones are looking at the trainee consulting (video or sitting-in), looking at records (problems or at random), discussing cases, doing tests (multiple-choice questions MCQs, modified essay questions MEQs, and self-rating scales), and finding out what other people think (partners, practice manager, nurses, etc.).

Self-assessment is an important component because it allows the trainee to look at his or her progress in ways and at a pace not determined by others. The methods available include self-rating scales; use is also being made of increasing computer-based instruments and other facilities such as the phased evaluation programme (PEP). This is a computer programme with MCQs and patient management programmes where the doctor can get immediate feedback on performance.

Educational assessment has to be an integral part of the educational progress, as described by Pereira Gray (1979). However, it creates a dilemma for the trainer. It is important to monitor and supervise trainees so that at every stage one knows how effective the learning has been and where it is going next. We have already pointed out that it is also part of the trainer's responsibility to ensure that patients get a good medical service. But the more responsibility that the trainer takes, the greater is the tendency for the trainee to become a passive partner in the exercise. By the end of the year it is essential that the trainee is fully in charge of his or her own assessment. Cummins (1990) has argued that helping learners to make continuous assessments of their own progress is important. Trainees then have to assume responsibility fully for what they are doing. Furthermore, they may well be more aware than the trainer of some of their personal deficiencies.

In practice, if the three-stage model described in Chapter 4 is adopted, the balance of control between trainer and trainee will change at the beginning of each stage, so that by the practitioner stage the trainee not only controls the learning but also the assessment. At that stage the trainee will want (and should be invited) to comment on the strengths and weaknesses of the training.

Effective learning

In this book repeated emphasis is given to the link between assessment and curriculum planning—the better the assessment, the better the learning plan. If trainers are not aware of their trainee's abilities in any great detail, how do they know whether the educational priorities are appropriate?

Example:
Michael came to the practice after 2 years as a registrar in obstetrics and gynaecology. He seemed very competent clinically and his entries in the medical records were good. On the surface it appeared that his consultations were good. It took Bill, this trainer, several weeks, however, to persuade him to accept a video camera in the consulting room. When Michael and Bill eventually watched his first series of consultations it became clear that in spite of good explanations at the end of his consultations, patients were never involved in decisions about their own health. After discussion about the advantages of this approach it was agreed to make this a high educational priority for the next few weeks.

Assessment enables trainees to look forward and to see their progress as time goes by. It enables them to see what they have achieved and where the next priorities lie.

Example:
Rachel joined her training practice after two post-registration hospital posts on the local vocational training scheme. It took her a while to understand the possibilities for the year, but as she and her trainer looked at her strenghts and weaknesses and developed a staged learning plan for the year, she became much more animated and enthusiastic.

Although it is convenient to think of assessment as involving a number of large-scale exercises looking at all areas, individual subjects or areas of behaviour can be tackled on different occasions so that the load for both trainer and trainee is spread. Assessment should be an integral part of many activities such as tutorials and projects and, as we shall see shortly, it should be written down at the time.

Characteristics of educational assessment

One of the problems for regional advisers and course organizers is ensuring the right balance between giving trainers too much guidance and paperwork, and no guidance at all. The former may either be ignored or, alternatively, followed slavishly without any thought. The latter leaves some trainers in the dark with no guidance.

The situation is similar to that facing those who write guidelines and protocols for managing clinical conditions. Other clinicians need to own the ideas in some way before they will use them, yet if they ignore important advice there is a real danger that patients get second-rate care (O'Dowd and Wilson 1991).

It is essential that when packages are produced everyone knows that they are properly constructed. A useful approach for advisers and course organizers is to list the important characteristics for assessment packages so that each scheme or practice can devise strategy and tactics within these guidelines. These characteristics are:

- A comprehensive framework of competence (i.e. a logical list of what the trainee has to be able to know or do);
- integration with learning and educational planning;
- agreed timing (related to trainee development);
- clear steps in assessment:
    clarifying objectives
    information gathering
    decision making
    recording
        giving feedback
        making plans;
- confidentiality;
- sensitivity to interpersonal issues;
- validity and reliability;
- feedback to trainer.

We will now look at each of these features in turn.

Comprehensive framework of competence

Chapter 4 stated that it is essential that trainers work out a logical plan of what trainees need to learn from each stage of the year (before they start negotiations with individual trainees).

The need to make sure that no major areas are missed out and that a correct balance is maintained between clinical areas (which are likely to dominate the trainee's thinking early on) and the other important topics has been emphasized. The challenge is to ensure that a logical framework covering knowledge, skills, and attitudes is used. One such framework is provided by the Oxford Region Priority Objectives (1988). Many people find it somewhat difficult to use, partly because it mixes together what general practitioners *do* and the *areas* in which they operate. So each trainer has to ensure that he or she has a master plan. In the second edition of the Oxford Region paper, the final chapter illustrates how one part of the region used the original objectives to devise an educational planner.

For this reason it may be easier in devising an assessment package to consider the separate components of the job under the headings described in the last chapter. This classification looked at what was *required* of a trainee (i.e. the attributes and abilities) in order to fulfil the *duties* of a general practitioner (i.e. content and context).

This is our preferred way, but there are others, such as the mutually agreed report system (Tibbott *et al.* 1990).

There is still a tendency for the clinical component to dominate learning in the general practice year. Skills in communication, organization, and management and medical audit are equally important. Moreover, once acquired they will last for life, unlike some 'facts', and since they usually receive proportionally less attention in the undergraduate curriculum and in junior hospital posts, they need to be emphasized in vocational training.

Integration with learning and educational planning

It cannot be stated too often that assessment and curriculum planning go hand in hand. Unfortunately, documents used for one often do not dovetail with documents used for the other. A properly designed assessment package will have the curriculum as an integral part, so that as comments, strengths, and weaknesses are recorded, and the learning priorities become immediately apparent. We show one such example in the appendix.

Agreed timing

Reference has already been made in the previous chapter to the fact that trainers may find it helpful to think of trainees proceeding through a succession of stages in the learning during the year. The new trainee stage is concerned mainly with safety and basic operations, the practising trainee stage involves everyday clinical practice, and the practitioner, stage audit, management, self-reliance, and continuing education. These stages cannot be standardized in time because trainees differ in ability. This means that assessment has to evolve as each stage is passed.

Example:
Susannah was a trainee with aboveaverage abilities. Because of her faster than average progress she and her trainer moved to the end of stage one three weeks earlier than average. This meant scheduling an earlier end-of-stage assessment and thereafter ceasing to monitor emergency care quite as comprehensively as previously. They moved to much more video consultation and using topic tutorials as a means of testing her breadth of understanding.

Although timing cannot be predetermined, it is helpful for both trainer and trainee to have a framework within which to operate. A possible plan might follow the follow the following scheme:

1. An initial assessment concentrating on personal circumstances and history, learning styles and previous medical experience, with a preliminary look at knowledge, skills, and attitudes. This enables trainer and trainee to identify basic strengths and weaknesses from which to negotiate an initial and overall learning plan. Some trainers use a specially structured intensive interview for this purpose.

2. Assessment at around 2 months which might seek to confirm competence in important areas of knowledge and practical skills while identifying broader issues for the middle part of the year as the trainee enters the *practising trainee* stage.

3. A further assessment at perhaps 8 months to check out previous omissions and lead into a plan for learning which will support the trainee's entrance into independent practice (or other career), with special reference to Stage 3 activities described in Chapter 4. This will show whether the trainee is ready to move into the *practitioner* phase.

It is important to recognize that while this framework incorporates major review and redirection points, much assessment will go on from day to day. Indeed, a great deal of the material used in the assessments at changeover between stages will be gleaned as the weeks go by: some of the ways that this can be done will become apparent in the next section of this chapter. The important thing is to have some means of recording day-to-day assessments so that later they can be retrieved easily.

The main purpose of this book is to help trainers develop effective formative (educational) assessment, but summative assessment (accreditation) sometimes gets in the way, as noted at the start of this chapter. One way round this is to use the assessment at the end of stage 1, if it seems appropriate, to tell the trainee that it is likely that certification or successful accreditation will be a foregone conclusion unless some major change in circumstances or commitment takes place, in which case the subject should be raised again. The main pass/fail aspect of summative assessment is then removed from the scheme.

Clear steps in assessment

Clarifying objectives

This relates to the comprehensive framework to which we referred to first.

Information gathering

Information must be derived from a number of sources, and from different types of assessment (for example, communication skills can be observed directly on video-recordings, discussed in conversations, and assessed by others, such as patients and staff). A variety of methods is already in use in different places and, in some, brief report forms are completed by those coming into contact with the trainee. The spreading of information-gathering both increases the likelihood of reliable judgements being made and helps to spread the burden.

The trainers need to learn a great deal about the new trainees in a very short space of time. Questions must be answered. What are their strengths and weaknesses? What are their attitudes and circumstances? How do they like to learn? Trainers must think carefully about what information they need at each stage and how they will get it. For example, as well as obtaining the information just mentioned for the initial assessment, information will be needed particularly about safety and basic clinical practice. So record reviews, case discussions, and MCQs will be helpful. Self-assessment questionnaires are also useful, because they involve the trainee and also give the trainer an idea of how much self-awareness can be relied upon.

Toward the end of the new trainee stage, other information will become increasingly important. How good are trainees at coping with everyday situations and problem solving? How do they relate to patients and staff? What are their attitudes to certain types of patients, such as the handicapped, those who always challenge the doctor, and bad appointment keepers?

Methods that will help here include video consultations, records and case reviews, MCQs, and discussions with staff.

Later on, in the practitioner stage, once the everyday work is managed competently, trainers will want to start thinking about such matters as audit and continuing education. A major change in assessment (and teaching) is needed here. Methods include looking at a project and what has been learned, exploring the care given by nurses and others, and discussions of published papers.

Example:
Mandy had done a project on auditing the care given in the practice diabetic clinic and Peter, her trainer, was impressed by the clear presentation and logical sequence in her report. Together they listed the good points—identifying the diabetic patients, an adequate sampling method for extracting the records, and a clear analysis sheet showing how many patients had glucose readings at acceptable levels. Peter was able

to point out to Mandy that next time she needed to look more carefully at published papers detailing where most shortcomings lie in diabetic care in general practice. He also commented that her solutions for improving follow up were somewhat unrealistic and that it would be helpful for Mandy to discuss them further with the practice nurse who ran the diabetic clinic.

Remember that each stage of assessment is both checking how far the trainee has got and setting the agenda for the next section.

Decision making

Once trainers have the necessary information they have to decide what it means. If a logical and structured approach has been followed, decision making is usually easy. However, it is necessary to consider what standard is appropriate for individual trainees and whether one is trying to achieve minimal, optimal, or ideal standards. This will obviously depend on the ability of the trainee and also on the stage that he or she has reached in the year.

Example:
In response to the introduction of the new GP contract, the local trainers' group decided to check through the arrangements for participation in, teaching, and assessment of child health surveillance. As a result, the trainers were clear about what the trainees should be able to do because the details were written down. Claire's trainee, Mark, was checked to ensure he could examine the hips of a 6 week-old baby and knew the primary immunization schedules, and Claire was able to decide how well Mark had done.

Rating scales are a useful guide to making decisions. The most widely used are those devised by the Centre for Primary Care Research, University of Manchester Department of General Practice (1988). Not only do they encompass the majority of important aspects of general practice, but they give guidance on how to judge a trainee's progress. There have been a number of modifications of the Manchester Rating Scales (MRS) and perhaps, seen from a contemporary perspective, more emphasis may need to be given to certain areas, such as understanding patients' ideas, concerns, and expectations, chronic disease management, and medical audit.

Trainers who do not use the MRS will need some other plan by which to make judgements about their trainees' performance. One option is to use the contents and contexts listed in Chapter 4 and examine each attribute and ability against each of them, as suggested in Fig. 4.1 p.40.

Recording

Unfortunately, all too often assessments are not written down. This means that trainers can avoid committing themselves, sharing the results, and having a detailed reminder of what conclusions were reached on an earlier occasion. Entering them in a training log not only gets round these difficulties but also identifies the priorities for the next section of the curriculum, thus stressing the link between curriculum and assessment.

Another recording method of assessment is a profile document. This shows the trainee's strengths and weaknesses from information provided by any number of individuals and at different times. It has been described by Bligh and Price (1991). Profile sheets can be completed and collected just like any other assessment document, and in this way a picture of the doctor is gradually built up. Hitchcock (1988) believes that this method has advantages in vocational training, including helping trainees to look at themselves as unique individuals, involving any number of teachers (consultants, partners, team members), improving communication between trainers and trainers, and motivating trainees to learn. All detailed and repeated written assessments should serve these functions.

Feedback

It is important that trainers should be able to give feedback sensitively and effectively. A good method is that described by Pendleton *et al.* (1984). In brief, it consists of clarifying any points that are not clear and then letting learners go first, in order to ascertain how far they are able to assess their own performance. Always start with good points and only later make recommendations for change, rather than criticizing. This approach can be surprisingly helpful.

Example:
Roger, who featured in a previous example, had done 6 months in another practice. He came with a reputation for being rather difficult, and it was apparent that the relationship with his previous trainer had not been very productive. It took a month or two to get him to discuss his feelings about what had happened. It transpired that his trainer had tended to go for the problem areas first, but had been unable to be specific about why things had gone adrift in consultations. After agreeing to a plan for looking at his videos, Roger became more relaxed and enthusiastic as Penny, his new trainer, always started with his strengths and was able to be quite detailed about areas for development, which included eliciting patients' concerns and sharing decision making.

Effective feedback should:

- be specific;
- be frequent;
- be close to the event;
- plan action.

Making plans

After each assessment it is important to agree further action to ensure that something happens.

Confidentiality

That written assessments need to be kept confidential is axiomatic. One of the excuses given by trainers for not writing assessments down is that they will contain sensitive and personal information. Doctors are used to handling such documents, however, and all that is needed is a clear set of guidelines. We suggest that the paperwork should belong jointly to the trainer and trainee, and the former should only release it to a third party with the permission of the trainee, unless there are overriding reasons. These include situations where the trainee's competency may be in doubt. However, it is also essential that visiting assessors to training practices are able to examine the paperwork for previous trainees, and non-identifiable past copies can be used for this.

Sensitivity to interpersonal issues

The question of confidentiality leads to consideration of the way in which trainers handle sensitive issues. Making detailed assessments helps to make the exercise more objective and less personal: trainers also need to know how to give feedback properly, as referred to above.

Validity and reliability

Proper assessment is time consuming and therefore it is essential that it is done as effectively and scientifically as possible. First, it must test the areas that it is intended to test. This is called *validity*. What is important (valid) is not just that the trainee *knows* what to do, but can actually *do* it.

Example:
Julie had answered questions about the injection of a shoulder joint prior to her carrying out such a procedure; she seemed very competent. When it came to actually doing the procedure, however, it became clear that she was completely unfamiliar with it. The assessment of her competence had been that of knowledge and not of her practical skills which were clearly deficient and needed to be tackled before she could carry out the procedure.

Secondly, if judgements are to be made about trainees they must be as accurate as possible. Another person (say a partner or practice manager) looking at a trainee's work on another occasion, should be able to come to the same conclusion. This is called *reliability*. The more people involved and the more aspects of a trainee's work examined, the more reliable the conclusions are likely to be.

Example:
Clare had been asked to do an MCQ as per of her initial assessment. There were three questions on paediatrics in which she did not score very well. However, when she was asked to do a further 12 questions her overall score was much higher, giving a much truer (more reliable) picture of her knowledge in this field.

Too much emphasis on reliability may, however, discourage assessment in areas where the doctor's activities are rather subjective or difficult to quantify. Equally, too much emphasis on validity may lead to a disregard for accuracy.

Example:
Tom had carried out a consultation with a rather anxious man which had been videotaped. He discussed it both with his trainer and with one of the other partners. All agreed that it was important that the relationship between Tom and the patient should be good since he would be seeing him again on a number of occasions. However, the two partners disagreed on how good it had been in this consultation. So they decided that they should view the next one to try to reach more agreement. In other words, viewing the tape was valid, even though they had not come to a reliable judgement about Tom's performance.

Feedback to trainer

The need to move towards equality in the trainer–trainee relationship has been stressed. This will be enhanced if assessment is not seen as a one-way process. Some assessment packages emphasize the need for the trainee to make a similar assessment of the trainer. But this may often be rather false. It may be better for assessment packages to include a section where the trainees give their views of the training rather than of the competencies of the trainers. This is recognized in the Mutually Agreed Report System. (Tibbett *et al.* 1990).

CONCLUSIONS

It is important that trainers are able to:
- distinguish between formative assessment and accreditation;
- identify their own difficulties with educational assessment and think of ways of overcoming them;
- use an assessment package that also incorporates the learning objectives and curriculum;
- make sure their package complies with all the appropriate criteria and that the results are written down;
- make sure their package fits with the three stages for the trainee year;
- be professional in their feedback: emphasize good points and provide specific help for the less good areas.

6 An environment for learning

In Chapters 4 and 5 the creation of a learning plan and assessment of progress was discussed, with emphasis concentrated mainly on the trainer and trainee. In this chapter we look at important features of the training practice and further characteristics of trainers.

THE TRAINING PRACTICE

Most regions emphasize the importance of the concept of a training practice. The following statement of principle is included in the introduction to the Oxford Region's *Criteria for the approval of trainers and training practices*:

Teaching practices and trainers are selected for the educational opportunities that they offer to their trainees. Trainees may learn from (a) experience and example working in the teaching practice, (b) teaching from the trainer, the partners and from other members of the practice team, (c) the other educational resources and opportunities available in the practice. All these must therefore be examined in the approval process.

(The document is reproduced in full in Appendix V see also Schofield and Hasler 1984).

First, we consider:

- Why a training practice?
- The training practice as a learning resource.
- Good practice and good teaching?

Why a 'training practice'?

Some people used to believe that one 'charismatic' teacher could teach trainees all that they needed to know. A view still persists in some quarters that training practices should not be special, and that trainees need to experience the rough end of practice to know what real life is all about. However, we have pointed out (chapter 2) that learners are heavily influenced by their environment, as well as anything the trainer may attempt to put across. if the environment and the teaching produce mixed messages, then the overall effectiveness of the teaching is diminished. When the tension is between 'Do what I say' and 'Do what we do', the latter is the more powerful message.

For trainees to get the maximum benefit from their training, therefore, it is very important that the training practice provides a high standard of care and is efficiently organized. These features exemplify and reinforce the messages of good practice that the trainee receives from other sources, such as reading or the day-release courses.

The other argument put forward against the development of high-standard teaching practices is that it produces an elitism that many other practices do not attain, and thus fails to prepare trainees for the real world. The riposte to this is that doing a job well should not be regarded as elitism. Trainees need to see general practice conducted and managed in an exemplary way, be it in city centre or leafy shire. Effective training for general practice should equip the trainees to cope with all types of practice regardless of social and economic circumstances.

The training practice as a learning resource

For a trainee to get the best out of training, a wide range of methods and resources should be developed (see Chapter 2). This is impossible for trainers to provide on their own as the range of knowledge, skills, and attitudes needed is enormous and cannot be encompassed by one individual. However, a training practice can provide this: each partner has different expertise, as do the practice nurses and health visitors. Many aspects of practice management and the organization are best taught by the practice manager and administrative staff.

Becoming a training practice is not a once-and-for-all transformation but a maturation and continual evolution influenced by many factors. These include: national and regional criteria for training-practice inspections, individual trainees, the local trainers' group, courses, and reading. The most important factor, however, is the motivation of the doctors and members of the practice.

Good practice and good teaching?

The development of a practice requires both the promotion of good practice and fostering of a good learning environment. In the rest of this section consideration will be given to satisfying both these requirements. This will cover various aspects of the practice:

- buildings;
- equipment;
- library;
- records and computers;
- partners;
- staff and teamwork;
- management systems;
- audit and quality assurance;
- projects and research;
- partners;
- the patients;
- the learning environment;

Buildings

The working environment is a major influence on how people feel about their job and how they perform. In industry, the Health and Safety Executive monitors poor working conditions, and multinational firms spend substantial amounts developing good working conditions for their staff. Why should not the medical profession give its working conditions the same priority? In some parts of the country circumstances make it difficult for a GP to influence working conditions and the effort needed to improve the building is great. The cost-rent system and the wish of many FHSAs to help improve surgery conditions should, however, make it possible for most GPs and their staff to work in conditions that enable them to deliver care of good quality. For an aspiring training practice the needs are greater—the trainees need space, ideally their own consulting room, but at least a room for reflective time and reading. Room is also required for meetings, computers, equipment, the team, and teaching. Extra consulting rooms for trainees are allowable under the cost-rent arrangements.

Equipment

There will always be debate about the newer or the more specialist equipment. Needs change continually and trends have to be monitored and appraised. A teaching practice has additional equipment needs over and above those of good clinical practice. For the trainee to develop his or her consultation skills it is important to have a video-recorder and camera. This equipment is useful for playing some of the excellent teaching videotapes that are available, as well as health education tapes for the patients. Other audio-visual equipment can also be very useful, particularly an overhead projector and flip chart for the practice clinical meetings.

Library

Keeping abreast of developments is virtually impossible without regular and selective reading. A collection of current journals, a selection of up-to-date reference books, and a choice of the wide number of books on general practice must be the core of the library of any practice that aspires to high clinical care, and certainly for those with trainees. It should be possible for trainees to refer regularly to current information, especially that related to general practice, and to read in depth about a specific subject that they might need to study. The teaching practice library therefore needs to be wider and better catalogued than that of a conventional practice. This can be achieved by the careful use of indexes or lists of useful references. Many trainers produce 'tutorial packages' of collected articles on specific subjects, such as that described in Hall (1983). The library of a teaching practice should also contain books and journals on teaching and learning general practice, so that all members of the primary health-care team can use them. If teamwork is truly to be encouraged, training practices should include literature from the fields of nursing, health visiting, and practice management, as well as medicine.

Records and computers

The emphasis on clinical records in teaching practices has been a disincentive to some practices wishing to start training and a cause of anxiety prior to inspection visits. The importance of clear, ordered records for good clinical care has often been lost in the sense of compulsion that many trainers feel. It is worthwhile remembering, however, that every patient is unknown to a new trainee who needs key information quickly. Good records are also essential for screening, audit, prescribing, and chronic disease supervision (Weed 1969). This is why the Joint Committee on Postgraduate Training for General Practice has laid down minimal criteria for records for training practices, covering ordering, repeat prescribing, etc. These national criteria have been supplemented by the requirements of individual regions. Meeting these criteria takes planning, time, and energy, which needs the commitment of doctors and staff. It has been shown that trained staff are able to order, summarize, and update the records to a very high standard (Zander *et al*. 1978).

Practice computing is developing rapidly. In response to the stimulus of the 1990 GP contract, the majority of general practices have a computer of one sort or another, providing anything from a basic age/sex register to a full system with a desk-top terminal for recording each clinical encounter. The number of doctors with terminals on their desk will increase over the next decade and trainees need to learn the tasks of data input and retrieval at an early stage.

Computers, used properly, have great potential to help in the improvement of clinical care. One of the most valuable functions of the modern practice computer is the identification of groups and subgroups of patients. Examples include the identification of clinical groups of patients (such as asthmatics, over-75s, the disabled), prompts to encourage screening (such as coronary artery disease, risk factors), monitoring of drug effects, etc. For a training practice the computerized records can be an essential teaching aid.

Example:
Peter wished to look at the identification and care of hypertensive patients in the practice. He first identified those patients labelled hypertensive. To check the computer, he listed all patients on hypertensive therapy, and found those who were not on the hypertensive list, but should have been. He was then able to find all those patients whose last recorded blood pressure was in the hypertensive range, but not on either list. These different ways of using the computer enabled Peter to produce a more accurate picture of those patients with high blood pressure and, at the same time, update and correct the information on the computer. Then, having

produced a true list of hypertensive patients, he was able to elicit information about various aspects of their care, including the identification of other risk factors, types and doses of medication, investigations done, and other associated diseases.

Many training practices already have a sophisticated computer system loaded with high-quality data. It would be very easy for the trainees to assume that this is the normal state of affairs. They need to know about different systems and how to introduce new computers into a practice. They also need to know how to keep the information up to date.

Partners

Trainees learn from their environment, which includes the people in the practice. At a minimal level, the other partners offer a model for the trainees and support for the training, which includes adequate time for learning and teaching. The trainee, after the first 1 or 2 months in a practice, creates space for the other members of the practice by taking a share in the clinical load. Hence, it should not be difficult for the partners to allow time, not only for the trainer and trainee to have uninterrupted tutorials, but for learning outside the practice, reflection, and individual work. The partners will have to consider their workload in terms of list size and out-of-practice work to accommodate the extra responsibility of teaching. Ideally, the partners should be actively involved teaching the trainee.

If all the partners do not see themselves as teachers then the trainee can miss out. The partners need to recognize the strengths and weaknesses in themselves and the others, so that the trainee can benefit from these strengths (see Chapter 2). If the partners are teaching, even in a limited capacity, the principles of effective teaching and learning are shared.

Staff and teamwork

The general practitioner works with an increasing number and range of people, and nowadays most people would agree that high-quality primary health care needs a team of people working together. It is essential to have the right mix of talents, with the appropriate training. The balance of skills may vary from practice to practice. In those districts where the community staff are not attached to practices effective teamworking is very much harder to achieve.

These different health professionals and staff need to work together with common aims to develop a team. Much has been written about teams and team development and there are excellent team development packages, such as the ACT Distance Learning Package (Munro 1992). Any trainer (in fact anyone who wishes to practice good medical care) must be aware of, and practice, principles of effective teamwork.

A training practice must not only have a strong and effective team, but the essential parts of that teamwork need to be overt. Trainees need to see and understand what makes teams work: this may not be immediately obvious. To use the example of practice meetings, the trainee needs to be able to attend, receive the minutes, and add items to the agenda. After the meeting, discussion of the process of the meeting with the trainer is essential learning—why a certain partner behaved in a certain way, why the ideas from the last meeting were not carried out, and why the meeting did or did not function well. A trainee can receive many other similar learning experiences from an involvement in the day-to-day working of the practice.

Part of team working that promotes development and enhances learning involves the team learning together. A practice can do a wide variety of things to encourage joint learning:

- Have team meetings with a visiting 'expert' to discuss a subject, e.g. the local obstetrician to discuss antenatal care, the local playgroup leaders to discuss care of pre-school children, the diabetic liaison nurse to discuss diabetic care in the practice.
- Involve all team members in the development of a joint protocol for the care of a patient group, i.e. the elderly, the terminally ill, asthmatics, etc.
- Create a practice journal club, with all members bringing interesting articles from their disciplines, literature for others to discuss.
- Form practice quality circles, with each group setting their own criteria and levels of achievement in different areas.
- Have joint tutorials in which, for example, the trainer, health visitor, and trainee discuss topics of mutual interest.
- If the health visitor is a fieldwork teacher, or the district nurse is a practical work teacher, it is possible to encourage the students to study issues together.
- Develop joint projects with team members: review access to the practice with the receptionist group, plan a health education programme for the mother and toddler group with the health visitor.

Management systems

Teamwork is important, but other activities also contribute to the efficient functioning of the practice. Most practices will have a system for repeat prescriptions, for receiving home visit requests, for out-of-hours work, without which it would be impossible for the practice to function. Often these systems are written down, so that all members of the practice are aware of what to do in certain situations. This may be in an office procedure book, or in notes for new receptionists. Other clinical and organizational systems at work in the practice are less obvious and are rarely written down, examples of these are communication channels or networks within the surgery, and the care of the anxious patient or the 'heart sink' patient. Leadership, too, is an important factor in change and long-term planning. The various leadership styles, need to be discussed between trainer and trainee.

For 'good practice', systems of organizational and clinical management need to be developed and perfected to help all the practice members to work effectively. For a teaching practice, these systems need not only to function, but to be overt and available, so that the trainee can understand how they are formed, how they work, well or badly, and how they can be improved.

Audit and quality assurance

Audit is being made an integral part of all general practice. The measurement by the practice of its standard of care, comparison of the achieved standard with an agreed protocol, and then making changes to deal with any deficiencies, is an essential feature of 'good practice'. It is very difficult, if not impossible, to practice to a high standard if one is not prepared to measure those standards and compare them with others.

For many years some practices have been measuring the quality of their work, e.g. their access, diabetic care, maternity care, immunization, etc., and sharing their results: some have appointed audit clerks to collect data. A few practices publish their results in the medical literature. Rather more practices include their audit results in an annual report. This allows members of the practice to compare results from year to year: it also allows others to be assured about the quality of some aspects of the practice, and helps planning of services for the future. At a more local level, groups of doctors and other members of the practice meet together, sharing the results of audits, and helping each other improve the quality of care.

For a training practice this striving for quality and the audit of clinical care is essential. Trainees will learn to measure the quality of their work as part of normal practice and establish patterns of behaviour that will endure for the whole of their professional careers. Like the systems of clinical and organizational management described above, the systems of audit need to be overt and clear, and must involve the trainee.

Projects and research

It is very difficult for a trainee to see research and projects as valuable if similar activities are not being undertaken by the trainer or other partners. It is important, therefore, if trainees are to be encouraged to do audit and research, that the members of the practice feel that these activities are important, and that they are part of normal practice. Projects are a useful way of expanding a trainee's thinking and understanding.

The patients

The patients in a practice are probably the trainee's greatest learning resource and the trainer can manipulate the trainee's case mix. The patients, too, benefit from being members of a training practice because of the required standards and the influence of young doctors coming each year.

Patients should be informed about changes of personnel, particularly the doctors, and this is often done by letter on the retirement of a partner and the appointment of another. In a training practice, this change is more regular and frequent and thus needs a different system for informing patients. The reception staff are key people who need to have guidelines about how to describe the new doctor and his or her responsibilities. The practice leaflet should have information about training, and the practice notice board or newsletter can play an important role in introducing the trainee to the patients. The difficulties attaching to the name 'trainee' and the implications of that word to the patients, staff, and doctors are discussed elsewhere. There are some aspects of training that have potential to interfere with patient care, such as the use of video in the consulting room, the sharing of visits to patients with long-term illness with the trainee, and the inspection of training practices. It is important that the necessity of these aspects is understood by the reception staff, so that they can explain in clear terms to the patients.

THE TRAINER

An effective learning environment needs as a basis a high standard of clinical care: the same argument applies to the trainer. If the trainee is told to practise one standard and sees the trainer practise another, it is the latter message which will prevail. The trainer, and trainer's development, may be considered under the headings:

- 'good doctors' 'good teachers';
- the scholarly trainer;
- the development of a good teacher:
    the personal picture of practice,
    professional teacher development
        teachers' courses
        reading;
- Development of extra-practice resources.

'Good doctors', 'good teachers'

Good doctors do not necessarily make good teachers. The following two examples may help to illustrate this.

Example:
Paul has been a trainer for 5 years. Recently, when he and his trainee, Pam, were looking at the subject of 'care of the elderly', he was able to offer a wide range of experiences, information resources, and methods that enabled Pam to understand fully and to practice the subject effectively.

He was able to identify patients that illustrate many of the points that he wished to make: independence of spirit, coping with handicap, the effect of the loss of a loved one, and the scope of community care. He was able to give examples both of cases that he had managed well and others that he had managed not so well. He could discuss with Pam his own difficulties and prejudices and explain the elements in his own background that could explain his behaviour. He was able to offer articles from the library that gave the arguments for and against elderly screening, thus allowing Pam to make up her own mind about it. He gave her a book about bereavement so that she might understand the problem more clearly. He suggested to Pam that she might go visiting with the district nursing sister to see things from a different perspective, and visit the local day centre and talk to the patients and staff.

Paul discussed the various aspects of these learning points with Pam so that she was able to sort out for herself the problems and joys of looking after the elderly and form her own management plans.

By the end of the discussion, the trainee not only understood Paul's approach to the subject, but realized that there is a wider spectrum of approaches. To be able to teach in this way, Paul has to be aware of how and why he practises and why he practises in his particular way.

Example: Derek has been a trainer for the past 8 years. In his early time in practice he was a clinical assistant in the geriatric day hospital. He also gave a tutorial to Gerry, his trainee, on the care of the elderly. Derek described the main elements of good geriatric care as he had always practised it and offered a number of tips to Gerry. But he had some difficulties in describing in detail exactly how he made decisions about patients (craft knowledge, see P.00). Derek based his package of care on that provided by the geriatric consultant 10 years previously, and which he had not questioned or updated: he was unable to identify recent papers on relevant topics. His approach to teaching is less likely to produce a questioning trainee who is prepared for the next 30 years of practice.

These examples show some of the added elements that are needed to move from being a good doctor to being a good teacher:

- Examine and analyse the features of practice.
- Identify the component parts and compare them with other doctors' practice.
- Pass on the information and skills.
- Personalize the information and skills to an individual trainee.
- Manage the trainee's education and use the other members of the team to extend this education.

It may be helpful to refer again to Chapter 2, and particularly to what we call craft knowledge.

The scholarly trainer

How academic should a trainer be, and what are the pros and cons to a learned approach to teaching general practice? The word 'academic' conjures up images for some that could be described as cold, pedantic, abstract, formal, and impractical. Whereas few would disagree that these are poor attributes for a doctor or teacher, it must be recognized that a learned and well-argued approach is essential and that many of the adjectives above are falsely associated with an academic approach. There are important elements in being scholarly, namely:

- being well read, with an ability to evaluate the literature critically;
- being able to retrieve relevant information;
- being able to present a reasoned argument based on evidence.

There are many trainers who do not feel that they need to be well versed in the general practice literature. They may justify their position by arguing that general practice is a skill based on experience, and that teaching should be from that experience. Others say that the field of general practice is so wide that it is impossible to keep abreast of the literature. It is possible to have sympathy with both of these points of view; while agreeing with the value of experience and the magnitude of the task of reading, it is impossible to be an effective teacher without a grasp of the general-practice literature. As we said earlier (Chapter 2), novices need to test their ideas against the evidence in relevant literature; therefore, teachers must be well informed rather than simply basing their teaching on personal experience alone.

The most immediate incentive for trainers to be scholarly is that it is virtually impossible to practise a high standard of medicine without being versed in the current medical literature. Regular reading is a difficult task for a busy general practitioner. So the skill of selecting and critically reading papers, journals, and books has to be acquired by all trainers in order that they can enable their trainees to do the same. The critical reading paper of the MRCGP examination seems to have been an incentive in this area.

Secondly, trainers need to set a good example: it is no good expecting trainees to read if trainers do not do it themselves. Finally, trainers should develop a broad academic base from which to teach. They are not only training doctors for practice now, but for the next 30 years. These doctors will need a broader range of skills to work in the twenty-first century—computing, management, communication technology, to mention a few. To be able to guide the trainees through this untrodden territory, trainers will need to increase the breadth of personal reading, into areas not previously considered applicable to medicine. Such reading can include literature in the world of education, both within and outside the field of general practice. This can be very stimulating without too much extra time and commitment. It certainly need not have those spurious connotations listed earlier.

Development of a 'good teacher'

Good teachers, like any professionals, have knowledge and skills made better by learning. Everyone can improve, although some find this more difficult to achieve than others.

The 'personal picture' of general practice

Each teacher needs insight and understanding of his or her own picture of general practice. Clarity of understanding of that picture comes from being able to identify the make-up of each detail, and where in the trainer's education and background that learning has arisen.

Example:
At a recent teachers' course, Thomas was asked to describe his personal view of general practice and from where it might have arisen. He chose to base his description on a series of articles, books, and writings, and then described how these were modified by the experience of meeting and discussing those ideas with a large number of people.

He said that his ideas of practice started with the solid base of his medical school teaching, which had been continually updated and modified by medical colleagues and reading ever since. His perspectives on the non-clinical aspects of general practice came from many sources:

- The psychological approach originated with the works of Michael Balint (1964) and Eric Berne (1964), but was modified and developed by contact with a management consultant, industrial psychologist, practice manager, and others.
- The approach to preventative medicine came from the RCGP occasional papers and other contemporary literature, but was modified by experience and by contact with a nurse facilitator, health education officer, and many others.
- The ethical approach to his practice came from a wide variety of readings, including Julian Tudor Hart's *A new kind of doctor* (1988) and McCormick's *Father figure or plumber* (1979), and was being evaluated and modified constantly by contact with colleagues and friends inside and outside medicine.

Thomas was able to describe in each area of his job, the content of that area, and the background that underpinned his approach to it. He was thus able to present his own 'personal picture', thereby enabling the trainee to develop one for himself.

This 'picture' might also be described as a shape or a list. Indeed, many lists have been produced to describe the content of general practice—the Leeuwenhorst document of European aims (*Second European Conference on the Teaching of General Practice* 1974), *The future general practitioner* (RCGP 1972), and the priority objectives of the Oxford Region Course Organisers and Advisors (1988).

The reader will have realized that it is difficult to define the content of general practice because there are very different opinions. Doctors will give different priorities to different subjects, reflecting a personal interest. However even though there may be disagreement at the boundaries, there should be general agreement of the core objectives of general practice;

without such objectives it is virtually impossible to teach (see Chapter 4). It is not satisfactory, therefore, to have a 'personal picture' of practice that is idiosyncratic and individual. The central philosophy must reflect the mainstream of general practice. Both doctors and trainers have continually to validate and reassess their picture of general practice with colleagues, either face to face or by reading, so the picture is continually evolving and developing. It is a dynamic concept.

Professional teacher development

The personal and professional development of trainers includes all aspects of medical education, with the additional requirements for teaching. Preferred learning styles are discussed elsewhere, and the range of learning varies from trainer to trainer. The developmental needs of a trainer are in the triad of:

- knowledge;
- skills;
- attitudes.

For specific development of teaching, the range of methods are equally broad:

- teachers' course;
- reading;
- trainers' groups.

Teachers' courses   The importance of courses in the development of a trainer cannot be underestimated. They provide opportunities for reflection about teaching, and facilitate the interchange of ideas and values between colleagues.

Most regions have a teachers' course for new trainers, where the contents can vary from the legal aspects of training to teaching communication skills, from educational theory to role-playing tutorials. It is an ideal environment for the trainer to acquire new skills and develop helpful attitudes. These courses can provide a good basis on which to start training, and equip new trainers to cope with their first few trainees. After a few years the trainer needs new stimuli and to develop new skills. Some regions respond to this by developing specialist courses for trainers, such as consulting skills training, teaching management skills, experienced trainers' course, curriculum planning, teaching quality in practice, etc. The Oxford Experienced Trainers Course is described in Appendix II.

Reading   As discussed already, regular critical reading is essential. There are now a number of useful books and journals for trainer development: many course organizers and regional advisers have lists of recommended ones.

Trainers' groups   The local trainers' group has probably the greatest potential, but unfortunately often the smallest influence on the development of the majority of trainers. Some trainers' groups play little part in the professional development of their members, with much of the time spent on administration. We discuss this in detail later (see Chapter 9).

Development of extra-practice training resources

Effective learning stems from a broad mixture of many experiences and situations (see Chapter 2). Other learning situations that are useful to broaden and diversify the trainee's experience are those outside the practice: the local pharmacist, the old peoples' home and day centre, the undertaker, the mental handicap team, the local hospice, the child guidance clinic, the local community hospital, the ambulance service, the FHSA, etc.

These resources should be developed, aims and objectives discussed and set, teaching methods clarified, and a form of assessment and feedback established. Inclusion of this list, with details of phone numbers and access, should be included in every new trainee's training log.

Although there are many advantages of a trainee being in one practice for the whole 12 months, for example care of chronic cases, developing relationships, involvement in the practice, there are limitations to the diversity of the experience. Many trainers get over this by arranging exchanges between training practices, in some cases visits to non-training practices, in contrasting areas and circumstances.

CONCLUSIONS

Summary

- The practice and its members are powerful influences on learning.
- Learners need a wide variety of experiences and approaches.
- Involvement of partners and other team members in the teaching takes careful planning.
- The practice should provide a high standard of care, and trainees need to understand how this comes about.
- Trainees need to think about their own approach to practice in some detail.
- Time and space must be created for the training.
- Roles, protocols, and practices relating to teamwork must be open and shared.
- Regular audit should be undertaken.
- Records and libraries should be of a high standard.
- Trainers need to use trainers' groups and courses and the literature of general practice to develop continually their approach to teaching.

7 Teaching methods

INTRODUCTION

So far, we have discussed what trainees learn, how their progress should be reviewed, and emphasized the need for training practices that provide high-quality care with a variety of teachers and experiences.

In this chapter various methods of teaching that make learning more effective will be considered. We shall look at factors influencing learning, and some of the points relating to adult and professional learning (see Chapter 2) will be discussed in relation to the training practice. Then we will consider some general approaches to learning (both new and old).

FACTORS INFLUENCING EFFECTIVE LEARNING

Single, static methods of teaching tend to become boring and learning becomes difficult. For effective learning there should not only be a variety of methods but also of different sources, contexts, and levels of abstraction, suiting the subject, the individual trainee, and the stage of development of that trainee (see also Chapter 2).

Trainees need a wide menu of methods of learning in order that they remain enthusiastic and interested. Too often, training becomes stuck in a uniform tutorial, lasting 1 or 2 hours each week, in which a clinical subject is discussed, often without preparation and with very little idea of how the subject fits into an overall plan. Both trainees and trainers need to choose methods from a *variety* of different options in order for the teaching to remain effective.

As discussed in Chapter 6, the practice will provide the basic *source* of learning, with all members of the team becoming involved on a regular basis. It may be helpful to compare the work of a GP with that of a trainer. GPs use the skills of fellow consultants: they are not expected to be skilled in neurosurgery or radiotherapy, but simply to have access to those who have these skills, so that they can use them when necessary. Of course GPs have to remain up to date in general terms about the development of medicine and relevant specialist activities. In a similar way, trainers should not expect to provide all the teaching themselves. They should constantly make use of other people and so widen the range of learning experiences. The term 'educational manager' rather than 'trainer' seems to describe this new role and indicates that it is possible for trainers to give up some of the traditional aspects of training in order for their training practice to develop. This will be discussed in more detail later in this chapter.

Learning needs to take place in an appropriate *context* for it to be effective.

Is the trainer's consulting room or house the best place for tutorials? It is logical to think of the issue under discussion and then match the environment to it. Sessions involving a great deal of referencing might be held in the postgraduate library. A session on management may best be held with the practice manager in her office. It is likely that other issues will be discussed outside the practice completely. The question to ask should be 'What location would provide the best environment for learning this particular issue?'

Learning takes place at different *levels* of sophistication and complexity, and if it is helpful relatively specific issues can be related to a broader plan. Trainers should try to match these specific issues to some kind of framework and, conversely endeavour to explain broad concepts by relating them to everyday practice.

Example:
Sally was halfway through her trainee year and had recently reviewed a patient with diabetes she had diagnosed 2 months before. Simon, her trainee, asked how things were going. Sally said that she was happy that the patient was on the right dose of oral hypoglycaemic drug and that her glucose level was in the acceptable range. However, she had had some problems in getting the patient to accept that therapy was necessary in the first place. She also had to keep reminding herself about the important complications of diabetes and how they should be watched for. Simon was able to point out that all these issues, and more, were relevant to many chronic diseases. Effective chronic disease management involves having methods of monitoring that remind the doctor and nurse what needs to be done, checking out the patient's ideas and concerns, and operating a proper repeat prescription system.

Subject

Learning needs to be appropriate to the subject. The method adopted is too often the one that the trainer or trainee is most comfortable with.

Example:
James was an enthusiastic, hardworking trainee, who was very keen to learn more about clinical issues. He attended lectures at the local postgraduate centre regularly and had a list of tutorial subjects that he felt were important for his early learning. It was only when he saw his own, and other peoples' videoed consultations that he saw his own lack of experience in communication. Thereafter he was able to discard his original agenda for learning and start to develop a more constructive one. He had not been aware of those particular needs, and certainly was not aware of that method of learning. He had been used to didactic lectures about clinical issues, but soon began to enjoy the discussions that took place around his and other videoed consultations.

Knowledge is probably best gleaned from reading books and journals. Skills need observation, practice, and feedback, while development of attitudes need directed discussion. The trainer thus needs to have a wide repertoire of methods to cope with the wide range of subjects.

Methods to suit the individual

Each individual has a preferred method of learning (Benner 1984) Some students regularly attend lectures and find them useful. Others never attend any, preferring discussion groups, case conferences, and personal reading. Everyone has an optimal time of day for learning: some people prefer lengthy tutorials, others prefer shorter, more numerous meetings. Teachers also have preferred styles and methods of teaching, and it is these that tend to dominate teaching/learning activities.

Example:
When Ann arrived at her well-organized practice she was given a practice timetable. This was unchanged from the previous trainee, and had been the same for many years. Her tutorial time was set for 8.30 a.m. She had always found that early morning learning did not suit her, and preferred to work late in the evening. When she proposed changing this timetable it caused considerable practice upheaval. The discussion that then took place highlighted the lack of negotiation that had taken place with all the previous trainees.

Honey and Mumford (1986) describe four types of learning style:

1. Activist style—learning comes best from new experiences, active involvement in work, and people. Learning is worst when the trainee has to be passive, has to theorize, and has to complete the task thoroughly.
2. Reflector style—learning comes best when student is able to stand back and think, and review carefully the task in an unhurried way. Learning is least accomplished in situations where the student is pressurized to perform, given limited data to perform, and is rushed.
3. Pragmatist style—learning is maximized when the theory and the job are obviously linked, where the task is practical, and the student has a chance to try out the techniques. Learning is low where it cannot be related to a practical task, is associated with no clear guidelines, and when there is no obvious reward.
4. Theorist style—the student learns best from being offered and using a theoretical model, can question and analyse the task, and deal in terms of concepts. The theorist-type student learns poorly when asked to perform a task without a conceptual framework, where the information is not organized, or is insufficient to form the basis of a logical conclusion.

Honey and Mumford suggest that courses and other learning situations should be investigated beforehand in order to ascertain that they are appropriate to an individual's learning style. The awareness of a trainee's preferred learning style can be useful for a trainer to encourage initial learning and enthusiasm for a subject.

The following points, based on a teamwork exercise, illustrate these different styles:

•   the theorist might wish to start by reading *Effective teambuilding* by John Adair (1986);

- the reflector would learn more by observing teamwork and discussing it;
- the activist might start with a joint audit project with the health visitors;
- the pragmatist might benefit from discussion about cases where teamwork has played a major part.

Although it is useful to be aware of a trainee's preferred learning style, the trainer must not confuse learning style with personality, and must appreciate that learning style is not fixed. Indeed, the trainer's role should be to help trainees be aware of their own learning styles, and to develop a wider range of styles to facilitate learning later on in their career.

One of the first books written about teaching in general practice (RCGP 1972) recognized four teaching styles:

- Authoritarian—tell and sell. The teacher makes the points and does not encourage questions because they will question his authority. This style is probably only good for conveying facts (but so is reading).
- Socratic—question and answer. The teacher always asks and the learner always answers, each answer triggering the next question. Information is only provided when the learner demonstrates an area of ignorance.
- Heuristic—find out yourself. The encouragement of learning by doing.
- Counselling—understand what is behind it. This is a less directive style than the others, with the aim that the learner shall understand the inter- actions that are taking place between him and the material being learnt.

Ideally a trainer should be able to use different styles for different situations.

Unfortunately, it is unlikely that a trainer will be able to work equally comfortably in every style. Byrne and Long (1986) showed that doctors found this difficult, and that moving from one style to another needed insight and an active wish to change on the part of the trainer. It is important, therefore, that trainers are aware of their own strengths and weaknesses as teachers and attempt to develop skills in the areas that do not fit with their natural inclinations.

If change is not possible, they can compensate for weaknesses by using other resources. This applies to knowledge and skills as well as teaching style.

Stage of training

The trainee's development will also determine the method and style that should be used for learning. 'New trainees' often have only been taught by rote and will not be aware of other methods of learning, finding a reflective style uncomfortable. However, they will, with guidance and encouragement, be able to consider a wider range of learning. Various pressures throughout the year may tempt a trainee into a 'narrowing' of learning: the trainer needs to be aware of these pressures and constantly strive to broaden ways of looking at situations. It would be inappropriate for a limited range of learning to continue during the 'practitioner' stage of training. By this time, the trainees should be encouraged to find answers for themselves and be aware of the uncertainties that GPs all work with.

Negotiation

Negotiation is defined as to confer (with another) with a view to compromise or agreement. Thus the individual curriculum is an agreed compromise at any one time, between the wants and needs of the trainee and the trainer's ability to meet these demands. This negotiation is a complex task made more difficult by the intricacies of the trainer–trainee relationship, the imbalance of experience of general practice, and the need of the trainee to be seen as a working member of the practice. These issues are dealt with more fully in other chapters. True negotiation requires both sides having access to the same information: in other words trainers have to provide full details about all aspects of teaching in order for trainees to have a choice.

To have a choice of method there has to be a variety of methods available. However, If the trainer is experienced in only a few, there will be enormous pressure in any negotiation (if ever any takes place) to use one of these methods. In many practices nearly all the teaching is the responsibility of the designated trainer, who is expected to provide a wide variety of methods. One way to extend the range of options is to involve other members of the practice team. It is the responsibility of the trainer to know who is best at teaching what, and who is best at a particular method; it is not the trainer's responsibility to do everything. There are, however, some fundamental skills that all trainers need, including clinical, communication, counselling, teamworking, management, and motivation skills. Negotiation, then, is not just about 'what', but also 'who' and 'how'.

Time

Time appears to be an abiding obstacle to effective teaching and learning. All trainers recognize the tension between time for patients and time for teaching, but the issue must be addressed. To learn effectively trainees must have time to think through new ideas, facts, and concepts they are being offered, and also time to understand, to question, to generalize, and to plan.

A work-based, apprentice style of learning encourages the doing, not the learning. Trainees are keen to emulate their trainers as soon as possible, without necessarily understanding what they are doing. In this setting learning occurs through assimilation. Unfortunately this does not encourage the thinking that is needed to see why something is done a certain way. This work-based mode of learning is good for gathering craft knowledge (what GPs do and why) and developing the skills of practice, provided that there is time for reflection. This need for time out is not often recognized by the partners within a practice, and the trainer may have to question the ethos that 'work is only seeing patients'. Indeed, it is not uncommon for trainees to say that their working week is too busy to permit private learning. Unless this value system is recognized and changed, the trainee will not feel able to take time out because the perception will be that proper doctors do nothing except see patients.

This reflection about the job will occur in various places, both in and outside the practice. The car journey to and from the day-release course plays an important role: trainees should not be expected to rush back to the practice to see patients.

Example:
Mark, a trainee, was very popular with the staff, as he was always up to time, could fit in a number of patients within his surgery without trouble, and, one day, completed the surgery of a partner who had been called out on an emergency, still finishing at the scheduled time. Appointments lasting 5 minutes seemed to be easy for him. Ann, his trainer, used the video-camera to watch his consultation techniques. In comparing the partners' consultation styles, he saw new methods and ways in which he could change. He was given permission to be late at the end of surgery, not to fit in all the extras, and to take time to think between patients. He became less popular with the staff temporarily but he acquired new skills and developed more satisfaction with his learning.

Preparation

Confusion arises for both trainee and trainer about preparation for learning. Trainers often state how difficult it is to get their trainees to prepare, or do any reading before a tutorial. Who should be preparing what?

Preparation is needed by both parties, but it is not necessarily the same for each. The trainee needs to find and organize material, so that new information can be discussed and related to the experience of the partners. Trainers, in the role of educational manager, require a different approach which includes both the needs of the trainee and considering also how best to provide the appropriate environment and method of learning. They do not need to be completely knowledgeable: indeed if they are, they may merely compete with the trainee, which is not the purpose of the exercise. If this happens, there is a danger that the trainee might switch off.

Example:
Stephen and his trainer agreed to prepare for a tutorial on the Mental Health Act. Stephen studied the documents and was able to quote the legal requirments for the use of each section. His trainer had found the records of a number of patients that had been selected to exemplify each of the categories and to highlight the problems that had arisen.

Educational management

A trainee's learning needs change and develop as their training proceeds. The content and the need for a range of methods will be overwhelming for a single trainer, and the need to involve other members of the practice in the education of a trainee has been emphasized already. Moreover, tutorials are not simply the filling-up of empty vessels with all the facts about medicine, general practice, and the nature of life.

What then is the role of the trainer? The answer is that the trainer becomes the 'educational manager' or 'coach', managing the learning resource of the trainee.

The term 'coaching' is well recognized in the field of sport. The name engenders thoughts of words like: skill development, support, encouragement, individual help, enthusiasm, guidance, words a GP trainer would probably like to be associated with. Coaching is also a term used in industry to describe the technique managers use to develop their staff to think and take decisions for themselves. Being coached can be described as: *someone working in a planned way under guidance to improve the quality of performance using the day-to-day work as a learning experience.*

In *The one minute manager meets the monkey* Kenneth Blanchard (1990) argues that the purpose of coaching is to get into a position to delegate. This description is compatible with the type of training that a trainee needs in the middle part of their training, when the 'practising trainee' is developing into a practitioner.

What are the salient features of coaching, and how can a trainer exploit these features to maximize the trainees' learning development? Coaching is the development of the trainees' *potential* by helping them think for themselves, thus improving their confidence in their ability to do the job. It needs a *plan* that fits into the individual curriculum that the trainer and the trainee have negotiated. The *opportunities* for coaching must be identified and used by both trainer and trainee. This applies to success as well as to failure. Effective coaching needs *risk-taking* on behalf of the trainer: important tasks need to be delegated so that the trainee can be stretched.

Example:
One of the greatest pleasures that Jack had in his clinical practice was the care of seven mentally handicapped adults in a residential home. He went once a month and reviewed their cases with the staff. These meetings and the subsequent consultations with the patients were a highlight that he strived not to miss. Janet, one of the residents, became sick when Jack was on holiday and saw Mary, his trainee, who continued to manage her after Jack's return. The staff at the home were concerned by Janet's condition and Jack and Mary decided that they would ask for a domiciliary consultation from a physician. Mary and Jack discussed the case and what they wanted from the domiciliary visit and agreed that Mary would attend it on her own. Jack hoped that he did not show his anxiety about this to Mary. When she returned they reviewed what had gone on and the care plan that was made for Janet. Mary had done well and had benefited from the experience in a way that would have been impossible if Jack had gone with her.

This example demonstrates the main features of coaching:

- identify the opportunity;
- brief the learner, negotiate and agree tactics;
- do it.

SOME GENERAL APPROACHES TO LEARNING

Access to craft knowledge

Much of the information that trainees require to practice is not the sort of knowledge that is found easily in textbooks or articles (see Chapter 2). For the trainee, it is the everyday considerations that enable doctors to perform effectively as general practitioners that are important, especially in the early stages of training. Conversely, the trainers often do not see these considerations as important and may not even be aware of the information and skills that they use to perform their job effectively. This highlights how important it is that trainers should be able to analyse their work and expertise if the trainees are to access the complexity of what is going on. It is not enough to be a good doctor, teaching requires discussion of not only what is done but also examination of how it is done. This is called *craft knowledge*.

Example:
Richard's first days as a medical student consisted of being taught how to take a history and examine patients. It took him at least an hour to go through the sequence of questions and examination before he came anywhere near deciding on a differential diagnosis. He was amazed by the speed, not only of the experienced consultants whom he observed, but also by the speed of the inexperienced house physician who seemed only a few years ahead of him. He was told to go through a systematic approach to history taking and then to examine all systems and record all his findings. In discussion with the house physician, he discovered that more experienced practitioners used a different method. It was suggested that he went through the next case with the house physician, to see and discuss each step in forming a hypothesis, and the questions used to confirm the diagnosis. The two of them then discussed other cases that Richard had clerked so that he could go through the same exercise.

Craft knowledge is what enables doctors to function effectively. To teach it to others one must:

- treat each case as unique;
- draw on experience more than textbook knowledge;
- take account of any specific circumstances and aspects;
- draw on an extensive repertoire of possibilities; and
- use analogies with previous cases.

Mastery learning

Much of the learning and teaching in general practice is concerned with coverage. Trainers have to cover the curriculum, testing at stages to assess that adequate understanding and competence is obtained. Some understandings and skills are so important that all trainees must reach competence. To teach these, another style may be more appropriate. Called mastery learning, it assumes total success.

Learning should progress in small steps, each easily made, and based on the assumption that each step will be successful as it will be based on previously acquired information and experience. Each successful step will provide the springboard to the next stage. This allows the trainee to remain optimistic and enthusiastic because the steps are manageable and there is a sense of progress. If the steps are too big, progress may be hindered.

There are five features of successful mastery learning:-

(1)   explicit, agreed goals;
(2)   prerequisite knowledge;
(3)   small steps;
(4)   assumption of success; and
(5)   early assessment and feedback.

Example:
When Jane started her training she was extremely anxious about being 'on call'. Madelaine, Jane's trainer, was therefore very careful to check that she had all the required information for her first evening on. Her bag was stocked and the telephone numbers listed. Jane spent her first few evenings on call at Madelaine's house, first watching and listening and then answering the telephone herself. Initially, they went to all calls together. Later, Jane would discuss the case with Madelaine when she returned: Madelaine would highlight how well Jane had performed. It only took a few weeks before Jane was happy to be 'on call' at home, with one of the partners covering in case of need.

Skills learning

The introduction of change is often made difficult by the lack of appropriate skills. For trainers these may include listening to trainees' agendas, exploring deeper agendas, and giving feedback. Trainees have parallel difficulties, lacking the skills to perform their new role as general practitioner. There are several stages to satisfactory skills learning.

1. Conceptual learning and modelling

It is necessary to make it clear at the outset why a new skill is needed. After a clear argument, it is helpful to demonstrate its use.

Example:
Early in Jane's training, Penny, her trainer, observed her consultations and perceived a lack of skill in enabling a patient to give information. Jane agreed that Penny's consultations seemed to flow better and the patients appeared more involved and subsequently more satisfied.

2. Deliberate practice and feedback

Having seen and understood the skill, it is time for the trainees to try it for themselves. It is important that they start on something easy. Feedback should be given to enable improvement to take place. Remember to:

- provide practice in simplified conditions;
- provide focus on specific skills;
- provide feedback from a credible source with similar ideas.

Example:
Jane and Penny initially used role play to enable Jane to try using open questions. Jane then attempted the same techniques in her consultations, which were recorded and analysed with Penny.

3. Automatization

Hopefully with enough practice the skill becomes ingrained and can then be performed automatically. Then it may be introduced into more complicated situations until it becomes part of expert practice.

4. Expert practice

Example:
Midway through Jane's year, in order to highlight her progress with Penny, they compared a video consultation that had been kept of her first week in practice with a much more recent one. The change in Jane's ability to obtain information was highlighted by both, and they were able to identify numerous skills that she was using, without thinking, to produce this improvement.

Cued modelling

However hard trainers try to minimize it, modelling will be the single most powerful aspect of the training year. The way in which trainers and their practices work will be an immense influence on trainees. It is the trainer's skills and attitudes that trainees tend to remember. Trainers need to be honest in highlighting their own strengths and weaknesses so that they can be explicit about the consequences of each and help trainees to learn positively from them. It is important that trainers highlight examples of good practice, while acknowledging instances of less good care (Berliner 1987). The relevant word is cue. Cued modelling enables the experienced trainer to harness the power of modelling, highlighting specific areas of practice.

Example:
Mark's trainer, Sue, wanted him to allow patients to take a more active role in consultations. She showed Mark the difference in their two consultation styles, pointing out her use of silence at the start of her consultations to give the patient

space. She highlighted the importance of the greeting, the setting of the consulting room, and the use of eye contact with the patient. Mark became enthusiastic about this change of style and it was agreed that he would record a further surgery in 2 weeks' time to analyse his attempts at this style.

Feedback

The special trainer–trainee relationship provides a powerful educational environment, one that many trainees are not used to. They have arrived from a medical education and hospital experience that does not generally provide one-to-one education. Reference has already been made to the importance of negotiation between teacher and learner, and to how ill-prepared for this trainees may be. There is a danger that trainees will take a passive role in the initial phase of training and allow trainers to dominate most of these negotiations.

Trainers would be quick to state that they learn just as much from their trainees, as the trainee learns from them. It is a privilege to be part of an environment in which learning is exciting. However, this environment often makes it difficult to provide the constructive criticism that is essential to trainee development. It may be helpful to review Chapter 5, in which factors that will help with feedback are discussed.

The most important simple thing to remember is that successful feedback always starts with positive points.

SPECIFIC METHODS OF LEARNING

The specific methods of learning may be divided into:

- learning from patients;
- learning from the team;
- learning from topics; and
- learning independently.

Learning from patients

Case discussion

Case discussion has always been a fundamental part of medical education and it is hoped that nothing in this book will have reduced its importance in the minds of teachers. It will remain the core of medical education, but it is important to understand the reasons for this, and to be aware of the dangers of relying on it too much.

For trainees, case discussion brings relevance to all the learning they do. It allows them to acquire new information and to work out new concepts acquired from other teaching. It enables both teacher and learner to use the first two stages of skills learning described earlier in this chapter. Case discussion also provides useful information about the trainee's performance and highlights areas of need for the future. Unfortunately, it tends to highlight only what the trainee perceives as important. Moreover, subjects appear in a random fashion, so it requires considerable organization for learning to be related to a basic curriculum. Some trainers, realizing both the attraction and potential weaknesses of case discussion, have a library of cases that they can call upon to widen the discussion in an appropriate way.

Problem case analysis

The trainee brings cases for discussion that he or she perceives as creating difficulties. This method is widespread and is still considered by some trainers as the only way of teaching. Properly done, it highlights the trainee's perceived needs. It needs little preparation, as the agenda is highlighted by the trainee and is stimulated by the problems that arise in everyday work. It is always relevant to current practice, is immediate, and often important. Because of this, trainees demand an answer quickly. Problem case analysis often takes the form of a call out of surgery, 'Can you come and help me through this particular patient's difficulty?' It is important that these exchanges are not lost. They need to be put into the context of other cases that have been seen and the broader concepts of practice that are being taught, otherwise simplistic solutions may continue to be used and the wider issues missed. Trainers must use imagination and keep the long-term goals in mind if this approach is to be exploited to the full.

Example:
Mark knocked on Jo's door between patients and asked if she could help him with a patient that he had in his surgery at that moment. This patient, seen by Mark on numerous occasions, had at last agreed that he needed some help with his alcoholism. Mark was unsure as to whether he should refer this patient to a psychiatrist, to a specialized alcohol unit for admission, or to Alcoholics Anonymous. After a short discussion about the problem, Jo was able to tell Mark about the local community alcohol team and he returned to his consulting room enthusiastically, planning to telephone immediately. After surgery, when discussing the cases that he had seen that morning, Jo and he continued the discussion of this particular case, highlighting the concepts of care that one needs to be aware of in dealing with alcoholics, referring Mark to some literature that he could read and some that he might like to give to patients at future consultations, and planning for him to continue his initial contacts with the community alcohol team with further discussions and a possible visit.
  Jo and Mark placed alcoholism on Mark's log as an area for further discussion, highlighting this particular case as one to follow up in the future.

Videos of problem case discussions between trainer and trainee reveal similarities between the trainer–trainee relationship and the relationship between doctor and patient. It is important with patients to explore the ideas, concerns, and expectations of their illness in each consultation. It is equally important with trainees to negotiate the problem in terms of the trainee's agenda. In practice, trainers frequently impose their own agendas, making assumptions about what the trainees want rather than asking how they need help. It is easy for the whole exercise to revert to an exchange of impressions and prejudices, with shared areas of ignorance being ignored. It is essential that these problem cases are put into the context of other areas of practice, that they are related to general concepts, and that the problems identified are used to make future plans for learning.

Example:
Stephen presented a problem case to his trainer, describing a hypertensive whose blood pressure was well controlled on beta-blockers but was keen to change treatment due to impotence. Although he described his anxieties about explaning the sexual problem of this patient, the discussion started amd stayed with the choice of drug that could be used to treat high blood pressure. At the end of the session very little discussion had taken place about exploration and treatment of impotence, and Stephen had to muddle through the next consultation with this patient.

Random case analysis

Random case analysis is a discussion of a case picked randomly from a normal surgery or visiting list. Neither trainer nor trainee has recognized any problem associated with the case prior to the discussion. Potentially rewarding, it is easy for the analysis to become superficial and fall into the same trap encountered in the problem cases, namely that of impressions and prejudices. It takes skill and persistence to develop each case so that maximum use can be made of it. It is important to delve beneath the superficial aspects to find others that are not fully understood or known. When conducted correctly, random case analysis is not only a very useful method of teaching but it is invaluable in assessment and curriculum planning.

Example:
Following his surgery, Tony brought his box of notes for a routine workshop. John, his trainer, decided to pick one set of notes from the middle of his pile. Tony described the case as a simple repeat prescription for oral contraceptives by a patient he had not seen before. The woman was not due for a cervical smear. He had checked her blood pressure, asked about any problems, and issued a prescription, the whole consultation taking only 5 minutes. During the discussion of this case, John and Tony ranged into the reasons for checking the blood pressure of young people taking the pill, at what age and how frequently gynaecological examinations should be performed, cervical cytology and target payments, the relationship between male doctors and young women requiring family planning advice, the use of a chaperone, and the advantages and disadvantages of having a dedicated Family Planning Clinic. They highlighted the need for a topic tutorial on family planning, and it was agreed this should be done by another partner who had particular experience in the area. This was written in the training log. John suggested that Tony should read Guillebaud's book (Guillebaud 1985) and that he should also make time to discuss with the practice nurse her role in family planning.

This example shows how the trainer exploited what appeared to be a simple consultation. It allowed the trainee to understand what would be going through an experienced doctor's mind during such an encounter (craft knowledge). It allowed the trainer to use the case as a means of discussing some key general issues (teamworking, organization, screening, etc.).

Consultation analysis

Consultations take up a large section of a GP's working life and cannot be ignored. Various ways of analysing the consultation have been described and details of these approaches have no place in this book. However, it must be emphasized how important it is for the trainer to have a clear framework in which to do this analysis.

There is clear evidence that skills of consulting can be improved. (Pendleton *et al.* 1984). Yet some trainers still feel uncomfortable about looking at doctor–patient interactions. This may be because very personal issues are discussed, or simply because the trainer lacks the ability to do it properly. Because of the delicate nature of some consultations, it is essential to follow the rules of feedback described in Chapter 5, and to seek the patient's permission. If the interaction is recorded on video, it must be used with discretion and stored safely.

Consultation analysis presents difficulties and traps for trainers, many of which are similar to those with other forms of case discussion. It is easy to have a relatively unstructured discussion about prejudices and impressions: hence the need for structure. In the book *The consultation an approach to learning and teaching* a list of tasks has been set out to enable the effectiveness of a consultation to be analysed (Pendleton *et al.* 1984). Roger Neighbour in his book *The inner consultation* sets out a slightly different structure (Neighbour 1987). The important point is that trainees need constructive and specific help, which highlights their strengths and makes suggestions for improvement.

The actual method used for analysing consultations will depend on circumstances. There are three obvious ways of doing it:

- sitting in;
- audio-recording;
- video-recording;

All have their champions, and all have their advantages and disadvantages.

Although a very simple method requiring no extra equipment or expertise, sitting in often causes great anxieties for the doctors, especially if they are trainees. It is also very difficult for the observer to remain outside the consultation.

Audiotaping is far less obtrusive and relatively easy to set up, but a whole dimension is missing. The trainer gets no view of non-verbal communication and therefore loses a lot of the advantages of visual methods.

Video is certainly the best option at present. It is less intrusive than sitting in, but provides both sound and vision. Video-recording remains a complicated exercise, however, and potential technical problems, especially those of sound quality, abound. The issue of anxiety in the trainee has been mentioned: one way of alleviating this anxiety is to share the exercise. If trainers start by video-taping one of their surgeries, it makes the exercise less threatening; some trainees may wish to view themselves in private first.

Trainees need to see in detail what they do and why (craft knowledge), and to have strong examples of good practice highlighted (cued modelling). Hence the need for trainees to see their trainers at work as well as the other way round. Observation of other experienced practitioners should be a fundamental part of training throughout the year, because some of the subtleties of practice will only become obvious when the trainee has acquired some basic experience. Unfortunately, in most training practices the trainee only sits in at the beginning of the year.

In summary, it is important, first, that trainers and trainees spend time looking at consultations, at what happens during them, at the clinical components, and at the attitudes and skills of the doctor. Secondly, trainees should have the opportunity of seeing not only themselves but also their trainers and other doctors at work, in order to see a variety of styles and skills of practice

Joint surgeries

In a joint surgery both doctors are part of the consultation. This is to some extent the antithesis of sitting in, in which the trainer tries to hide in the corner of the room, observing practice but staying out of it. In a joint surgery, there are opportunities for both trainer and trainee to observe practice.

Example:
Anne and her trainer hold a joint surgery weekly. They watched one of Anne's recent videoed consultations and agreed that she was unhappy with her style of opening her consultations. During the next joint surgery Anne's trainer showed her a number of different options for greeting and welcoming patients, following which Anne assumed the role of lead doctor and practised similar methods. Between each consultation, discussion took place about the method used. From this Anne was able to decide on a number of styles she would use in the future.

This example illustrates one use of joint surgeries, which is to enable the trainee to experiment, with the trainer present as back up. But as time goes by the balance of power will alter, the trainee taking more responsibility.

Many trainers who use this particular method of teaching also highlight its advantage in passing over cases from trainer to trainee, in order to balance the trainee's workload. Chronic cases that might otherwise be difficult to transfer to the trainee can be handed over during a joint surgery. Alternatively, it is possible for trainees to bring problem cases to this event for advice and discussion. Negotiation will be needed if these surgeries are to be fruitful as it is important that both parties know and understand what is expected of them.

Workload and learning

In the current arrangements, most of the trainee's time is taken with acting the role of general practitioner, and it is easy to forget that he or she should still be learning, even when not supervised, overseen, or taught. The danger is that some trainees will simply want to do the job because being a doer is more attractive than being a learner. The opportunity to become autonomous as soon as possible is highly alluring (see Chapter 2). This is confirmed by trainee comments on their training year at Oxford—seeing patients is the most popular activity. Indeed, there would be cause for concern were it otherwise, as trainees have 30 years or more of seeing patients in front of them. Nevertheless, this enthusiasm for doing the job can impede learning the job.

There must be a balance between theory and practice. It is too easy for trainers to see their trainee as another partner, taking on commensurate responsibilities and workload. Too much theory becomes irritating, but too much practice will result in the trainee simply learning how to get by rather than grasping underlying details and concepts. Trainers need to look carefully at what is right for each trainee at the different stages of the year, making sure that there is time for messages and ideas to sink in.

Schon (1983) in his book *The reflective practitioner* emphasizes the importance of learning in practice. The professional learner has a greater need for practical experience than for practical knowledge. Time needs to be given to reflect on each new situation as it arises to make the most of the learning opportunities, matching these to other experiences.

Striking the appropriate balance between a trainee's workload, and the amount of time for learning and teaching is one of the challenges faced by every trainer. Trainees need experience of common conditions in general practice, and need to develop the ability to manage them with an economy of time, but with repetitive clinical conditions the amount of learning will diminish. Ideally, the trainee's exposure to this kind of work will also diminish. Unfortunately, the evidence from a survey of trainees' clinical workload suggests that this does not happen (Hasler 1983). This survey found that the trainees' workload was static after the second month and was related to the workload of the practice rather than learning need.

The trainer, in the role of educational manager, needs at times to expose the trainee to being busy and coping with the pressures this creates, but at other times the trainer needs to protect the trainee from those pressures, to allow time for learning and reflection. Trainees will need guidance on how to use this time, and how to manage all aspects of their time in the practice.

Trainers need to be aware of the trainees' changing needs. Most recognize the early need for survival, the support that trainees need in their first few weeks, the need for discussion about each case, the reassurance that needs to be given about each problem. As time goes by the trainees' workload can be increased, new concepts can be introduced, and they can contribute more to the operating of the practice. Trainers should be aware, however, that even later on in their training it is not necessarily right that trainees should always be seen just as a competent pair of hands. Which is more important for trainees in their last few months? Another surgery containing more sore throats and earaches, or time to finish a project or to appreciate some of the intricacies of audit? Another diabetic clinic, or time with the practice manager and the district nurse to discuss the formation of such a clinic?

Finally, it may be helpful to identify ways that learning takes place when performing the job:

- learning from experience;
- reflecting on that experience;
- practising skills previously learned;
- seeing the consequence of previous actions;
- putting ideas into practice;
- learning by doing; and
- coping with the stress of everyday work.

Learning from topics

This is what most teachers and learners understand as teaching in its formal context. Whereas the types of learning activities reviewed previously are generated largely at random, topics, by their nature, are chosen specifically.

While the timing for any particular subject may be stimulated to some extent by situations that arise in the course of routine work, it is important that they relate to the curriculum agreed between trainer and trainee and reflect the results of educational assessments. Discussion should reflect both the immediate needs of the trainee and the broader, long-term needs. Whatever the subject, it must be taught in a way that suits the individual trainee.

We have emphasized that it is not necessary, or even desirable, that trainers should have the skills needed to do all these tasks themselves. Other people, such as partners and team members, can contribute to this process. Sometimes whole topics will be delegated; on other occasions it may only be aspects of a larger issue. It is also useful if some of the teaching sessions involve more than just trainer and trainee. Indeed, in comments on training practices, trainees frequently say they wished they had had more input from people other than their trainer.

The face-to-face contact between trainer and trainee, discussing topics that have been agreed as important by both, has always been perceived as a tutorial. What is a tutorial? Each trainer has a different answer to this question, and there is a danger that their approach becomes standardized regardless of trainee or topic. One way to stimulate new thinking about its effectiveness is to look at video-recordings of tutorials in the light of the task list in Chapter 3. A common problem is that the trainee's agenda is not clearly identified and assumptions made by the trainer may be quite wrong. At the end of each tutorial, notes on trainee performance should be recorded and plans made for the future—another task that is often neglected. Further stimulation and variety may be introduced by having other team members conduct tutorials.

At the beginning of the year, the time the trainer and trainee spend together will be directed toward helping the trainee become clinically competent, and the method and content will reflect that need. Towards the end of the year, tutorial time will be used in a different way, with the trainer helping the trainee develop learning patterns and resources in other parts of the practice or outside.

The form of the tutorial needs to be tailored individually to the needs of the trainee, in a similar way as the subject matter. As the trainee's educational needs, learning style, and experience develop and change, then the construct of the teaching will need to change, and thus the time for teaching/learning will be used differently.

The task list for effective teaching and learning (see Chapter 3) will help both trainer and trainee to understand and negotiate the process that will enable learning to take place. Thus the role of the trainer in the tutorial varies and develops from teacher to educational manager. The speed and consistency of this development will vary from trainee to trainee, and also according to the current needs of the trainee and the ability and skills of the trainer. Both trainees and trainers need to be aware of the demands on their time together, and be flexible in their approach to that time.

As educational manager, the trainer is also responsible for the learning climate within the practice, both in its broadest sense as a teaching practice (see Chapter 6) and in the day-to-day running. The trainees need space to learn, this means physical space with creature comforts and free of interruptions.

Learning from the team

In describing the trainer as 'educational manager', frequent reference has been made to use of other members of the practice, and their role in the trainee's learning. Staff, medical and non-medical, have an essential part in the trainee's learning and development. It is important that the trainee establishes a relationship early on with all members of the primary health-care team, and many trainers have a set pattern of sitting in and visiting with everyone for the trainee in the first month. The relationship that the trainee develops within the team can be varied, to meet his or her educational needs and wants.

As teachers

Other partners can offer skills and knowledge that the trainer does not have; and the health visitor, practice nurse, practice manager, secretary, and receptionist also have unique skills and knowledge that the trainee can utilize. These other practice members need encouragement and support to develop their role as teachers.

As models

The trainee learns from the theoretic background, practising, and modelling from peers. Thus the role of every member of the practice is important as a model, and if the members are able to explain why they behave as they do and what their potential is, the learning that the trainee obtains from the practice can be maximized.

As co-workers

The trainee can learn a great deal from working closely with members of the practice team: a case study and conference with the health visitor; drawing up a job description and planning the appointment of staff with the practice manager; co-counselling with a community psychiatric nurse, etc.

As co-researchers

Research and audit need to play a large part in training if trainees are to be encouraged to think critically. They could look at the quality of asthma care with the practice nurse, research weaning difficulties with the health visitor, look at local resources for the elderly with the district nurses, or research the quality of access to the practice with the receptionist.

To test out the trainee's concepts

Adult learners need continually to confirm or refute concepts that they have about their jobs. Trainees, as well as using their peers at the day-release course, can use all members of the practice to test their concepts, to get a broader view of general practice. These roles will vary from trainee to trainee, and throughout the year with the same trainee.

Effective teamwork is a prerequisite for delivering high-quality primary health care. Trainees need to be able to work effectively within these teams. Some, of course, will be 'naturals', requiring very little for the development of their skills, but others will require considerable help. Trainers therefore need to be aware of what constitutes effective teamworking skills, and to provide an environment in which the trainee can become more proficient in these skills.

Much of the time the difficulties that trainees will come across will be to do with process and not task. It is important that trainees understand this and are able to analyse relationships within the team. A detailed discussion of group dynamics is not appropriate in this book, but two of the issues that appear to be important may be identified.

Roles

Many ways of looking at group roles can be helpful. Belbin (1981) described a number of important team roles that people in groups tend to adopt. It is useful for trainees to be aware of the roles that they and others play, and to be able to discuss them. This analysis should enable them to recognize the roles needed to enable teams to function effectively. They can also try out new ones for themselves, to provide a greater repertoire for the future.

Leadership

Organizations need leadership if they are to adapt and survive. For instance, who should be the leader of the primary health team? Is it necessarily the senior partner? This and similar issues need to be addressed, and the trainees should be able to try out their own leadership skills.

Observing the activities of the primary health care team will provide trainees with an opportunity to consider these issues. Their role as outsiders is one that they are unlikely to be able to take on again. It is possible to watch the group at work, the changing roles of the members, the leadership issues that arise, the games that are played within the group, and to analyse how all these factors help or hinder the work of the team. Analysis of these processes may enable trainees to avoid the traps that await any new partner in practice.

Example:
James was a trainee in a four-partner practice. He attended all the practice meetings and was encouraged to express his own views whenever he felt they were appropriate. He was puzzled about the difficulty that the practice was having in introducing a screening programme for the elderly. It appeared to him that it was a simple task that could be shared equally between all members of the team, and he expressed this view quite forcibly during one business meeting. He was surprised that his input was not helpful in reaching a solution. Later he discussed this issue with his trainer and attempted to analyse what had happened. He had not been aware of the underlying tensions between district nurses, health visitors, and doctors about whose responsibility it was to perform this contractual task. The senior partner and the long-established health visitor had never seen eye to eye about their own roles, and the former's rather domineering attitude did nothing to improve matters. Following this discussion James was able to take a back seat at the next few meetings, describing subsequently to his trainer what he thought was going on. He developed a clearer view as to why this task was not as simple as he had first thought, and was able to discuss

other ways to break the deadlock, coming forward with a suggestion of lobbying and bargaining, which he now realized could be very important in practices.

Independent learning

Under the present arrangement of medical training, only a very small proportion of an individual's professional career has any organized learning. What happens when this structure is not available? We know that some knowledge gained at the outset of one's career may change twice before retirement, so there is a great need for regular updating. We also know (from experience with the introduction of the 1990 contract) that it is equally important to evaluate and re-adjust attitudes and the roles that doctors play in response to the needs of the profession and society.

To do this, trainees will need to develop skills to find information, critically analyse that information, recognize its importance, and relate it to their environment. The academic background of medical school and university may not help them in recognizing useful information in the professional environment of practice, as the needs of each are different.

In this section we will discuss the methods of learning that can be useful in the early years of training to enable the trainee to develop the skills required to maintain competence throughout their career:

- critical reading;
- projects;
- case studies.

Critical reading

The traditional method for professionals to remain up to date has been reading, and a mass of journals is available to doctors, seemings to increase each year in response to this thirst for knowledge.

How does the doctor, and particularly the young doctor, choose the journals to read? It would be impossible to read them all. Disappointingly, many appear to read little, relying on contacts with other doctors and brief summaries from the medical 'newspapers' to maintain their knowledge. The introduction of the critical reading paper in the MRCGP examination has increased the importance to trainees of critical analysis of papers and journals. Hopefully, this skill, once developed, will enable them and encourage them to continue reading throughout their life. Shared reading and journal clubs, both in practice and within the trainee group, can encourage those who do not read systematically, at the same time helping them to analyse the value of specific journals.

Up to now we have not mentioned books, although much of what has been said applies to them equally well. The volume of information and the speed of its change has meant that books have become less important in maintaining professional knowledge, as the information they contain becomes out of date very quickly. Despite this, their importance remains, and trainees need to be encouraged to use them to develop the skills and attitudes needed for good practice in areas that are not subject to the same speed of change.

Teachers should remember that the models their trainees see in professional practice are likely to set a standard for them throughout their career. If they see learning by reading as an important part of their training practice, they are likely to continue.

Projects

Project work is a fundamental part of learning about practice and should not be confused with research. Activities in modern general practice depend on abilities that can be learned from organizing and completing a project.

Trainees need to have experience of:

- gathering and analysing information;
- organizing information;
- relating new information to established practice;
- changing established practice.

These basic skills are needed for introducing change, but many more equally important skills will be developed by the completion of a project:

Communication skills	Personal communication
	Presentational skills
Management skills	Time management
	Personal organization
	Teamworking
	Problem solving
	Objective setting
	Questioning
	Completing/finishing
Leadership skills	Motivating
	Delegating
	Supporting others
Audit skills	Forming protocols
	Reviewing the literature
	Critically analysing information
	Organizing data

Why is it that so few trainees undertake projects when one sees this impressive list of skills that can be developed from such an activity?

1. Many trainers introduce the idea of projects very early within the training year. Sometimes this happens even on the first day, when the individual trainee agenda is focused on the more immediate problem of patient management. As discussed in Chapter 4, the 'new trainee' is still in an

early stage of training, when project work is not seen as a priority. A project should be part of the 'practitioner' stage of training and used to develop the individual's ability to work independently.

2. Projects are time consuming and get in the way of other learning activities that appear more important to the trainee. Even when introduced in the later stage of training, they compete for time with patient care, finding a practice, the MRCGP exam, and, last but not least, the pressures of home, which may include a new marriage or small children. However, projects need not be complicated and time consuming. Answering a simple question can be just as useful as a complicated activity, and is more likely to be finished. A structured approach to project work can help the trainees to manage time more effectively. Each stage is set out specifically with an expectation that it will be completed by a certain date (Table 7.1).

3. Many projects are imposed upon a trainee by the needs of the training practice. 'This would make a good trainee project' is often heard at practice meetings, when no one else is prepared to take it on. Once again, we emphasize the fact that the trainee's agenda is likely to be the deciding factor in whether an activity is undertaken or completed. The project must be seen as an important part of his or her learning, and he or she should choose the subject.

It is not necessary to leave it entirely to the trainee, trusting to luck that he or she will see the importance and find a subject. As most course organizers know, trainee projects seem to take place regularly in certain practices and not at all in others. This is no coincidence, as those practices that undertake projects themselves set a model to which most trainees respond. There is also likely to be a list of subjects awaiting the enthusiasm of a practice member, or trainee. This provides a choice for trainees who are unable to find their own subject.

The reason for project work in training is to develop individual trainees' skills, which they will need in independent practice, and which we have listed above. Most projects will be practice-based and may never be seen outside. They do not need to be original or published. If trainees feel that their project needs to be original and published, most of them will never pass stage one of our structured approach (Table 7.1). This does not mean that the same rigours do not apply, or that they should not use the same expertise and technology.

Case studies

We described the role of case discussion in medical education earlier in this chapter. Little has been done to develop this to the extent that has occurred in other disciplines. The training of health visitors and district nurses has included case studies for many years, and much can be learnt from their experiences.

Table 7.1 Potential time course for project completion

Time in weeks	
1	Choosing a project
3	Planning
	reading
	discussing
	organizing
6	Obtaining information
10	Collating information
12	Analysis
13	Presentation

This method requires the trainee to study a case in depth, looking not only at the disease and its diagnosis but also at the relationship between the patient and surroundings, the doctor and the primary health-care team, the patient's family, and society. Medical teachers have tended to limit their use of this method to studying the theoretical background to a particular case, researching the literature, and writing a critique of the subject. The nursing and health visiting teachers expect their students to then explore the social aspects by interviewing the patient, and others in the family, to explore the understanding, impact on, and feelings of each. This requires the trainee to look carefully at all aspects, and then write it up. It enables the trainees to:

- research a topic that is clinically based (and therefore related to day-to-day practice);
- explore the roles of other team members and decide how the whole team can be more effective in providing care;
- understand the impact of disease on the family;
- organize and present their work;
- receive formal feedback.

Trainer and trainees could benefit from joint activities in these areas with health visitor and district nurse trainers.

TRAINING LOGS

The importance of recording assessments was emphasized in Chapter 5, in which the concept of the training log was introduced. A nautical analogy may be helpful—a log should tell people where they have been, where they are now, how that has been determined, and the course that is set.

It should also be borne in mind that occasionally ex-trainees (including those who are blameless) appear before the General Medical Council (GMC) or in court, and trainers may be asked for detailed information. Without written records, trainers may find themselves in difficulties. The overriding reason for keeping training logs, however, is to help make teaching and learning as professional as possible.

Reasons for records

Doctors spend a great deal of time and effort in maintaining adequate patient records, so it should not be necessary to argue the case for this activity. Training logs are equally important for the following reasons:

1. The fallibility of memory. Just as GPs cannot remember all the salient points regarding their patients, so trainers cannot remember all the details about their trainees. It is important that recording takes place close to the event so that nothing important is forgotten. This enables trainers to refer back and recognize patterns of behaviour that might otherwise not be noticed.
2. Need for continuity and coherence. Involving all members of the team in teaching requires good communication between those concerned. Trainers need to know what the trainee has learned from other people and what those people's assessments were. For their part, trainers need to communicate their overall strategy to others involved in teaching, so that a consistent approach is maintained.

Content

The construction of a training log will vary from place to place. Some regions have developed packages for this purpose. Whether to impose such packages (which makes it difficult for trainers to 'own' them) or to leave trainers to devise their own (and risk them being incomplete) presents a dilemma. Whatever their format, however, logs should contain information about all aspects of training.

Information

A great variety of items can be recorded, most of which are obvious. This list is not exclusive and is intended only to illustrate the possibilities:

Basic information:
- curriculum vitae
- job description
- timetable
- study leave

Learning experiences:
- patients seen

- chronic diseases
- emergencies
- case studies
- situation experiences
- audits
- projects
- teaching methods used
- meetings with team members
- clinics attended
- books and articles read
- practical procedures carried out

Decisions made

This section should show conclusions and decisions that have been made. It includes the results of assessments and conclusions from teaching sessions. For example:

- analysis of strengths and weaknesses identified from the selection interview;
- completed Manchester Rating Scales;
- consultation rating scales;
- conclusion of mid-term assessment and other assessment reports;
- personality tests.

Plans

In this section the information from the previous two sections will be used to make plans for future learning. They would consist of specific issues that needed to be highlighted and discussed, preparation that would be needed to be made for those sessions, and the methods to be used in the session itself. It is helpful to have both short-term plans and longer-term plans which would be recorded in less detail. These plans should be related to the original curriculum (see Chapter 4).

Ownership

Ideally, a log should be a shared record of the teaching and learning, with access afforded to all members of the teaching team, information being placed in it at the time of each educational activity, and information obtained from it in planning future activities. It is an integral part of training and would be the basis of the trainees' education, not only during their training year, but for their whole career. It acts as an *aide-mémoire*, for the trainer and for the trainee, holding all the information in one place. Clearly, there may be sensitive information, and the question of who owns and has access to this part of the log is important. At certain times there may be information that it is not appropriate to share with others. If necessary, this part can be held separately. It is important, nevertheless, that all except confidential information about teaching should be held within the main log, and that all those involved with the teaching should contribute to that information and be able to draw upon it.

At the end of the training year, it is hoped that trainees will see it as a valuable description of their training, with important information for the development of their future career. Much of the information will also be important for trainers. It is an important description of teaching and will be needed for their reapproval. When used for this purpose, it is quite simple to remove identification so that individual trainees remain anonymous.

Example:
Short-term plan
After a discussion of a case of a patient with depression, the plan could be 'The trainee to look up information about the new antidepressants, and we develop together a policy for antidepressant therapy in the next tutorial.'

Example:
Long-term plan
After filling in a rating scale and discussing the priority objectives, the trainer and trainee feel that the trainee needs to develop an awareness and skills in the area of teamwork and team development. The entry in the training log might be 'Develop an understanding and skills of teamwork. During the next 4 weeks the trainee should complete the following exercises:

1. Read chapter in *Management in General Practice* by Pritchard *et al.* (1984).
2. Read *Teamwork* by Vincent Nolan (1987).
3. Observe:
   (a)   practice meetings;
   (b)   monthly psychiatric team meeting;
   (c)   the working relationship of the practice nurses and the doctors in the practice, and discuss with the trainer the processes involved that enhance and inhibit teamworking.
4. Organize a joint project with the health visitors, midwife, and the doctors to formulate a practice policy on prenatal care. In 4 weeks time we will review progress in the area of teamwork and make another plan.'

CONCLUSIONS

In this chapter we have tried to present a wide range of educational methods which will help trainers to broaden their approach. We suggest that they should:

• use a variety of methods involving differing sources and contexts, relate detailed points to general concepts;

- use appropriate methods to suit the subject, the individual trainee, and the stage of training;
- negotiate regularly for methods as well as subjects;
- allow time for the trainee to not only do the job but also to learn to do the job;
- prepare for learning (trainers and trainees do it differently);
- explain in detail what you are doing (craft knowledge), remembering that it is difficult to find this kind of information in textbooks;
- help trainees to develop and rehearse effective skills (mastery learning);
- emphasize good models of practice (cued modelling), give feedback that is skilful and sensitive, identifying strengths and then weaknesses;
- develop teaching expertise within the primary health-care team to provide a wide choice for teacher and learner to suit the individual's needs;
- encourage trainees to develop into independent practitioners with appropriate methods of learning.

8 A developing relationship

The personal development of trainees is closely interconnected with their medical and professional development. We have already referred to the advantages of staging the trainee year (see Chapters 4 and 5) and the difficulties that adults may have in learning and doing at the same time (see Chapter 2). In this chapter we shall look at the personal growth of the trainee and at the trainer–trainee relationship, two closely interrelated subjects that can be sources of extreme joy and misery. These issues will be examined from the point of view of both trainer and trainee: we shall also examine the trainee's relationship with the practice. The purpose of this chapter is to challenge ideas and offer insights to all those trainers who have, at one time or another, felt strong emotions of any sort about their trainees or about their training.

THE TRAINEE

Many trainers, trainees, course organizers, and regional advisors have a problem with the word 'trainee'. It does not conjure up the image of a mature doctor with at least 3 years postgraduate training who shortly could be responsible for the medical care of a registered list of patients. The name originated in the 1945 NHS Act and has resisted subsequent attempts to eradicate it. Suggested alternatives have included Registrar in General Practice, Assistant in General Practice, and Doctor attached to General, Practice, but the term 'trainee' persists. The name is unhelpful and can be seen as pejorative. However, the important issue of the debate is not what name is used but how the trainee is treated in the practice by doctors, staff, and patients, and how trainees perceive themselves.

The trainee as an individual

In a practice that has been training for a number of years, with a fixed system of working and a planned programme of education, it can be tempting to consider each trainee as a clone, to be fitted into a practice pattern, with a fixed timetable, planned curriculum, and standardized teaching methods. But the teaching should be personalized to each trainee in order to optimize learning.

The trainee must be recognized as an individual, with a personal background and culture, particular learning needs and styles, and with unique motivation. These individual characteristics need to be explored and understood by a trainer so that the training can be personalized. This may be difficult for trainers because of their own background and experience, which may obscure open and objective appraisal of each individual trainee.

Good trainees/bad trainees

The terms 'good/best' or 'bad/worst' are often encountered in trainers' descriptions of trainees. What do the trainers mean by these terms, and what is it that makes them describe their trainee in this way?

Often, the origin of these professional judgements relates to factors other than the performance of the trainee. These ancillary factors include:

- the attitude and expectations of the trainer;
- the circumstances of the practice;
- the personal characteristics of the trainee—and the wisdom of making professional judgements on personal characteristics.

Example:
Murray approached Janet 4 months through his trainee year, saying he was unhappy with his training, and asked if she would take him on for his second 6 months. Janet said that she would have to speak to his present trainer first. The phone call with Murray's trainer was revealing: he described a man who was not willing to be taught, not motivated to work properly, did not understand the basis of general practice, and was reluctant to discuss subjects of importance—an obviously 'bad' trainee.

Because Janet liked Murray and felt he had potential, she agreed to take him on for the rest of the year, albeit with trepidation. She found him very willing to learn and widely read in the GP literature. He was eager and wanted to take a fair share of the work but let her know if he felt maltreated. He was clinically very competent and teaching sessions did not need to concentrate on physical disease manifestation and treatments.

It transpired that Murray's previous trainer had had a fixed programme of tutorials on clinical subjects, and was of the opinion that trainees were there to be told what to do. It is not surprising in these circumstances that Murray was labelled as a 'bad' trainee.

Example:
During the 12 months that Jennifer was in the practice, new premises were built and occupied, a partner resigned and was replaced, and a woman partner took maternity leave. Bob, her trainer, had a difficult time with Jennifer. She was always demanding his attention and was critical of the quality and quantity of tutorials. She was reluctant to take on any extra work and was described as lazy and uncooperative by another partner. She seemed to get closer to the nursing staff than she did to the doctors and thus appeared distant.

After she left, and as life in the practice settled down, Bob realized that a major part of the view of Jennifer—as a 'bad' trainee—was related to what was going on in the practice rather than with her as an individual.

For trainers to fully understand their trainees, they must first be aware of those feelings, prejudices, values, and circumstances that affect their own judgement. A trainer must also try to separate those feelings that come from the personal characteristics of the trainee from judgements of the trainee's professional merits.

Understanding the trainee as a person

The trainee's needs are both the driving force and a limiting factor in the teaching. It is vital, therefore, that the trainer be aware of and understand these needs. This understanding is the first stage in gaining insights into the prejudices and blocks that inhibit awareness. There are two techniques that most trainers use, either consciously or subconsciously, to help them understand the trainee.

The first is to obtain a full CV. The second is to have the trainee spend a large amount of time during the first few weeks either sitting-in or visiting with the trainer. This allows time for mutual understanding, personal negotiating, and 'bonding'. Often a conflict arises because the trainee has to develop a wider circle of contacts with the other partners, practice, and community staff. In practices where the trainer does not allow this time for the trainee to settle into the practice, the trainer–trainee relationship can often be difficult for many months to come.

A third technique is now being used by some trainers to reach a greater understanding of their trainee's personal agenda. This is a long interview of the type used in selection interviews in industry. It contains questions on a wide number of areas, many of which most trainers and trainees rarely enter. An example is given in Fig. 8.1.

However, a grave disadvantage is that the process is very one-sided and yet again the greater power of the trainer is emphasized. It behoves a trainer who wishes to use this technique to be aware of its hazards, and to attempt to minimize them.

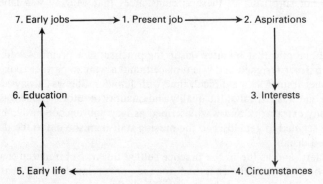

Fig. 8.1 One example of a selection interview (reproduced by permission of Kaisen Consulting Ltd, Bristol).

THE TRAINER

We have already stressed that it is very important for a trainer to be aware of his or her own personal agenda and circumstances.

The trainer as an individual

The basis of much teaching comes from the trainers' previous experience, which influences their effectiveness and outlook.

Example:
Jane, an enthusiastic ex-trainee, was keen to get started herself as a trainer. Unfortunately, her enthusiasm was not matched by that of her first two trainees, who were poorly motivated and both chose not to follow general practice as a career.

Jane become disheartened and her enthusiasm waned. She therefore expected less of her subsequent trainees. Fortunately, her third trainee was bright and responsive, but it took him many months to change the prejudice that Jane had developed about training and trainees.

Roger Neighbour in his book *the inner consultation* (1987) warned about the effect of one difficult patient on subsequent consultations. Trainees need to guard against a similar phenomenon.

Trainer personal development

The professional development of a trainer is discussed in chapter 6.3 and, as with trainees, trainers' personal development should parallel their professional progress.

Both trainers' courses and trainers' groups should help trainers to gain insight into their attitudes and values, and to develop skills and knowledge. The training practice itself should afford a similar opportunity (see chapter 9).

Modelling: the costs and benefits

Many experienced trainers will have noticed that the trainees seem to grow more and more like their trainers, and that each training practice will beget trainees with many similar behaviour patterns. The concept that trainees grow more and more like their trainers, that is the 'trainee models the trainer, was excellently described by Freeman and Byrne (1982).

This phenomenon has been referred to already in Chapters 12 and 6. There is no doubt that modelling does occur, and it can create problems: the solutions are awareness of the possibility, and the use of other resources to fill in the trainee's gaps. This includes exposure to others to allow the trainee a breadth of experience.

Example:
Simon is a trainer: he is a gentle man who at times seems unaware of his surroundings. He doesn't use a diary, instead making notes to himself on his hand or on scraps of paper. He is inevitably late for meetings, surgeries—in in fact, all appointments. His partners tolerate this weakness because of his affable nature.

Unfortunately, the trainees from his practice, because they are mainly working on 'Simon time', develop the habit of turning up late for appointments. This produces annoyance and frustration among doctors, patients, fellow trainees, and course organizers alike, and is likely to get the trainees into deep water when they enter practices that operate on Greenwich Mean Time!

To avert such problems in future generations of trainees one or more things have to happen:

- Simon has to develop time-keeping and diary-keeping skills and arrive at the right place on time.
- Simon has to be aware of his weaknesses and encourage and cajole his trainees to be punctual, i.e. do what say, not what I do.
- Simon and the partners in his practice need to be aware that time-keeping is a subject that needs to be assigned to another partner, who will help the trainee develop the appropriate skills.

There are many other examples of trainees acquiring bad habits from their trainers: lack of critical reading, workaholic tendencies, laziness, poor attention to administrative work, limited appreciation of the wider concepts of practice, etc. Trainers need to be aware of these gaps in the trainee's learning and manage their teaching accordingly. But there may be times when modelling is appropriate and it is often helpful if this is 'cued' (see Chapter 7).

Teaching style/learning style: possible conflict

Both the trainer and trainee have a preference for certain types of learning and teaching. Learning styles, and the implications for the trainer, are examined in more detail in Chapter 9. Much has been written about teaching styles in general practice (RCGP 1972; Byrne and Long 1973) and how different trainers have a preferred style of teaching. Clearly there could be problems in a situation where the style preferences of trainer and trainee conflict.

Example:
John is a widely read trainer who enjoys theoretic arguments and discussions about any subject. He would be described as a Socratic teacher: that is one who is highly informed and encourages his trainees to derive their own answers to problems using their own reasoning processes. He expects the trainees to ask him about problems but rarely offers solutions.

Richard, John's trainee, is enthusiastic about general practice because of the close patient contact. His spare time is taken up with car maintenance and DIY. He is a pragmatist and needs to be doing to learn.

The conflict between these two is obvious; Richard has no time for the theoretical, head-in-the-clouds way of John's teaching, while John perceives Richard as a non-thinking artisan verging on illiterate. It needs a lot of insight and flexibility to prevent John and Richard's relationship disintegrating under the strain of this conflict in outlooks.

The disabling of trainers

It might not seem possible to trainees, who perceive their trainers as rock-like and confident, that trainers can often be disabled by their trainee, i.e. that the trainer is unable to function effectively and the trainee's learning suffers as a result. Such disability can arise as a result of any one of a number of things, several instances of which are presented below.

The situation of the ex-senior registrar

'What can I teach him? He knows more than me', is a familiar reaction of a trainer on examining the CV of a new trainee. The trainer can only see the trainee's areas of strengths, not the deficiencies. A more objective view will allow the trainer to identify areas of need and an agenda for learning.

The trainee who has no wish to continue in general practice

This situation includes the doctor going into a pharmaceutical company and the prospective parliamentary candidate. The trainer must ask himself, 'What am I doing here?' or, more positively, 'What can I hope to do here?' This might help to start the negotiations for shared aims for the trainee's time in the practice.

The trainee about to enter a relative's practice

There is a temptation for the trainer to feel that the trainee wants to be prepared for only one type of practice and that this is a difficult task. The trainee in this situation can benefit greatly from a broad look at practice, which allows new ideas and techniques to be brought into the established practice.

Falling in love with/lust for a trainee

Until recently this subject had not been aired, and the problem is probably more widespread than most trainers would care to acknowledge. The brave article by an anonymous trainer (Anon. 1990) describes one such instance. The guidelines for avoiding reoccurrence of the situation are laid out by the author:

- Tutorials should be conducted in normal working hours with other people in the building.
- Meet socially only when spouses or other suitable people are present.
- Do not attempt to help a trainee with personal problems that have no bearing on their training.
- Stay in touch with your own feelings about the trainee.
- Talk to someone at an early stage of inappropriate emotional involvement, and arrange early separation.
- Remember that the course organizer and regional advisor are there to help.

Collusion about areas of weakness

It is very easy in a developing relationship for both members to be less than honest about areas that they both find difficult. If this situation continues, the trainee may leave the training practice with those weaknesses never having been discussed and remedied. An effective assessment package, with honest self-appraisal and feedback, can help overcome these problems.

Postgraduate exams

There has been much debate about the disruptive effect of the MRCGP. Many trainees also take the Diploma of the Royal College of Obstetricians and Gynaecologists and the Diploma in Child Health in their trainee year. These exams can greatly alter the trainee's agenda for learning, and training may be disrupted for a long period of time. It requires honest negotiation at an early stage and an understanding by both parties of each other's needs. As far as the MRCGP exam is concerned, insights into the curriculum of the exam and the needs of the examiners would enable both trainer and trainee to realize that the two learning agendas are not dissimilar.

Being an effective trainer is a difficult, time-consuming, but very rewarding task. Most of the difficulties and rewards of the job are associated with the long and close relationship of trainer and trainee. The qualities required in a trainer to develop and maintain this relationship may be itemized:

- Awareness—awareness of self, of values, attitudes, of strengths and deficiencies, of preferences and dislikes: awareness of the same characteristics in the trainee.
- Honesty—honesty of feeling follows on from awareness, and is, in turn, followed by honesty of expression.
- Flexibility—the trainer needs to be flexible enough to cope with a wide range of trainees and their needs. This requires: a wide range of skills within the trainer and practice, and support from many sources, including the practice, the trainers' group, the course organizer, and home.

THE TRAINER–TRAINEE RELATIONSHIP

The authors of '*The future general practitioner*' (RCGP 1972) comment of the doctor–patient relationship that:

The making of this relationship depends on rapport, an emotional element, and communication, an intellectual one. Both of these, of course, are two-way exchanges . . . The relationship between doctor and patient therefore requires both rapport and communication. Without the good relationship the gathering of information, the defining of problems and the proposing of solutions are infinitely more difficult.

These sentiments are equally valid for the relationship between trainer and trainee. Having earlier considered the two protagonists separately, it is now appropriate to look at aspects of the relationship between them:

- power and status, including gender issues;
- development over the year; and
- establishing and enhancing the relationship.

Power and status

The use of the words 'power' and 'status' in the context of the trainer–trainee relationship is anathema to some trainers, as are statements like 'We are all equal in our practice' and 'Our trainee is treated the same as the partners' to others. It is essential to be aware of and overtly recognize that there is inevitably a status difference between learner and teacher. The more obvious aspects that illustrate this are:

- the trainee often has to have a reference from the trainer;
- the trainee is temporary;
- the patients in the practice are the 'trainers' patients', or 'partner's patients'.

Further evidence about the perceived status of trainer and trainee comes from research carried out by Paul Arntson from North Western University, Michigan, USA, while on sabbatical at Oxford in 1983. He wanted to study the difficulties, that trainers and trainees perceived with their relationship, and he asked all the trainers and their trainees to complete a questionnaire about the potential and real value of many of the training activities that they did together. Two extracts from his report are: 'Trainees view their role in the relationship as being more passive than the trainers expect it to be' and 'Both the trainer and trainee felt that the trainees should be more active in the tutorial.'

This latter perception was repeated time and again in the study. The trainers wanted the trainees to ask more questions, interrupt more, refer to the literature, and make general conclusions from specific cases.

To say that the trainee must be more active questioning and challenging does not diminish the trainers' and course organisers' responsibilities for changing the situation. One must be careful not to 'blame the victim', the trainee here. From the trainee's perspective the freedom to challenge and think independently is new, time consuming, and potentially very dangerous. Trainees have rarely been given such freedom previously, their patient responsibilities take most of their time, and there are no perceived rewards for challenging people in authority while potential sanctions appear everywhere. It is one thing for a high status person to say that it is alright for he or she to be challenged. It is quite another thing for anyone else to believe it.

Ways of diminishing the difference in status are considered below.

There have been several publications about issues of power and status between learners and teachers. In their book *A practical handbook for college teachers* (Fuhrman and Grasha (1983) introduced the concept of 'psychological size' and this seems to have relevance to the trainer–trainee relationship. They described psychological size as the ability that one person has for helping or hunting others. People who are perceived as psychologically 'big' have a high potential for influencing and controlling other individuals. When one party is bigger than the other it interferes with open dialogue between the two of them. The authors felt that teachers can increase two-way communication and reduce their own psychological size in the classroom by avoiding:

• ridicule and sarcasm;
• punishing remarks;
• an overly formal manner;
• discouraging, disagreement;
• a display of overly complex knowledge;
• one-upmanship.

The transactional analysis in concepts (Berne 1964) of parent adult: child is often used in the context of the doctor–patient relationship. At any one time in the relationship either individual may be said to be exhibiting the feelings and the behaviour characteristics of one of three states of mind, or 'ego states'. These are:

• the parent—who commands, directs, prohibits, controls, and nurtures;
• the adult—who sorts out information and works logically;
• the child—who produces intuition, creativity, spontaneous drive, and enthusiasm.

These three ego states play an important part in everyday life, and together they are thought to represent the complete personality. According to transactional analysis, each person exhibits one of the above in any conversation, but can shift from one state to another with varying degrees of ease. People still tend to respond appropriately to the offer or stimulus of others. For example, an adult stimulus is likely to produce an adult response and a parental stimulus is likely to produce a child-like response. The same concept is valuable when looking at the trainee–trainer relationship and the same conclusions remain, namely that an adult : adult relationship is the healthiest and most functional of the various permutations.

Development over the year

Frequent reference has been made to the fact that trainees develop considerably over the trainee year in their needs, wants, and experience. Their teaching/learning has to respond to this change. Trainees, as well as maturing clinically over this time, also mature emotionally. They develop from a senior house officer (SHO) or registrar with limited responsibility to potential partners with custody of the health of about 2000 people.

This emotional development over the trainee year has been likened to the maturation from child to adult, and many trainees remember with some feeling the adolescent time of their traineeship.

Example:
Rebecca was one of the brightest and enthusiastic trainees that James had ever had. The year started with a lively exchange of ideas, and she absorbed the concepts and practicalities of general practice like a sponge. She soon became a competent doctor with her own list of admiring patients. However, after 4 or 5 months things seemed to go wrong. At one time she felt that James was being too directive in the tutorial and then the next that he had not prepared enough. One day she had too many patients and the following day complained that receptionists were not allowing her patients to see her. James used to go home feeling as though he had been through a wringer. He didn't know how to make it right and after a while gave up trying.

Slowly Rebecca became more satisfied with life. She resumed her project, and prepared it for publication, and also restored her close relationship with the staff, which had become strained. The tutorials took on a new life as they discussed articles she had read and audits that she had done. By the end of the year they had mutual respect for one another. James and his wife see Rebecca and her growing children on a regular basis.

As well as her obvious skills as a doctor, Rebecca was an accomplished artist and produced a painting for James that described the turmoil that she felt in the middle section of the trainee year. It was called *Each year is different and so is the next*. The pattern across the print became confused and turbulent and then settled into order and structure. The colours in each quarter were different but the pattern remained the same each year.

The emotional turmoil illustrated in Rebecca's picture was also demonstrated in Paul Arntson's survey. He found that there was much greater disagreement between trainer and trainee in the middle third of the year than in the first or last thirds.

The transition from dependent through counter-dependent to independent is demonstrated in the training of many professions and crafts. The pattern is repeated in the progress of the naval officer cadet, the articled solicitor, the apprentice plumber. Roger Lipsey in his book *An art of our own: the spiritual in twentieth century art* (1988) describes the development of the artist from apprentice through journeyman to master. In the chapter entitled 'Joys of the apprentice, sorrows of the journeyman' he writes: 'The journeyman is neither a child nor an adult, neither joyously tied to the mentor nor wholly free. A dark time ensues.'

Recognition of this transition, and the trials of the trainee passing through it, is a critical act which opens the way to a solution. The educational importance of recognizing this transfer from dependence to independence, from child to adult, is touched upon in Chapter 2. In many cultures there are 'rites of passage' to mark this event. This transition is rarely recognized in vocational training, however, and trainees often have to work out for themselves where they are. It helps to make explicit the understanding that the trainee will develop and that the relationship also will change and mature over the year. This change will vary in both degree and pace from trainee to trainee.

Sometimes it is possible to recognize this transition in the training year—the trainee acquiring his or her own night-visit bag, a mid-term assessment that recognizes the transfer to the practitioner stage (see Chapter 5), or, at least, a verbal statement that the trainee will get his or her accreditation form signed.

Establishing and enhancing the relationship

Throughout this chapter we have described features that work against the development of an effective relationship and some that can enhance the relationship.

An effective trainer–trainee relationship needs:

- self-awareness;
- honesty and openness;
- mutual respect;
- sharing each other's values and goals;
- being useful to each other.

We have already pointed out that it is difficult for the trainee to be responsible for the development of the trainer–trainee relationship. It is much easier for the trainer to be more objective and take the greater part in the maintenance of an effective relationship.

In *A practical handbook for college teachers*, referred to earlier (Fuhrman and Grasha 1983), the authors offer four suggestions for increasing the involvement of the students:

- creating a conductive physical environment;
- taking student goals and needs into account;
- establishing class norms which encourage involvement;
- eliciting feedback from the students.

Fuhrman and Grasha recognize the importance of the learning environment in establishing and maintaining the relationship. In a similar vein, Kelly Skeff (Skeff *et al.* 1988), who visited Oxford in 1987, emphasized this point, and listed several features of an effective learning environment:

- Stimulation:

    show enthusiasm for topic and learners;
    show interest through body language;
    use animated voice;
    provide a conductive physical environment.
- Learner involvement:
    look at learners;
    listen to learners;
    encourage learners to participate;
    avoid monopolizing discussion.
- Respect comfort:
    use learners' names;
    acknowledge learners' problems/situations;
    invite learners to express opinions;
    state respect for divergent opinions;
    avoid ridicule, intimidation, interruptions.
- Admission of limitations:
    acknowledge learner limitations;
    invite learner to bring up problems;
    admit own errors or limitations;
    avoid being dogmatic.

At first these points may appear obvious and a little naîve, but inspection of videoed tutorials will often reveal that trainers fail to be aware of many of them. The only way to be sure that these guidelines are followed in tutorials is to observe them directly, using video, and get feedback.

This last point is a reminder of the importance of regular skilful feedback and the disabling feeling that develops when it is not forthcoming; the openness of a good relationship that encourages the giving and receiving of honest feedback. If a trainee receives regular updates from the trainer on his progress, the anxiety that might otherwise arise is lessened.

In Paul Arntson's study, referred to earlier, the author suggested three activities that might demonstrate to the trainee the trainer's intention and desire to have a more equal relationship:

- discussion of the trainer's videotaped consultations;
- discussion of videotaped tutorials;
- joint research projects on topics that the trainer has little expertise on.

Thomas Harris in his book *I'm OK, you're OK* (1970) described and set an aim for an effective relationship based on the concept that the most effective relationship was one that benefited both parties. For both members to optimize their relationship they need not only to recognize their own and others' wishes and needs, but also to express them in a way that is helpful and non-threatening. This is the difference between aggression, passiveness, and assertion,

The trainer–trainee relationship is like any relationship, needing insight and honesty to establish and maintain it. Marinker 1981) has written, 'For the trainer–trainee relationship to be effective, both must be prepared to look at that relationship with some courage.'

CONCLUSIONS

- All trainees are individual and their needs and personalities must be clearly understood.
- All trainers must be aware of their own attitudes, values, and prejudices.
- Trainers need to be aware of why some trainees might render them ineffective.
- Trainers must be aware of their own perceived power and status, their trainees' emotional development, and how they can enhance the trainer–trainee relationship.

9 Vocational training schemes

INTRODUCTION

A great deal of activity is organized outside the training practice to provide education, support, and administration for both the trainer and the trainee. This activity can be very varied, depending on whether the trainee is on a three-year fully integrated scheme or a one-off trainee year: the frequency and length of course activities will also be relevant. In this chapter we examine all the important aspects of vocational training schemes, with the exception of the hospital posts which are the subject of Chapter 10.

The vocational training scheme (VTS) covers both activities and people and includes the day or half-day release course; the trainers' group; the course organizer; the postgraduate centre; and sometimes the regional advisors and associates. All these play a role in the effective education of trainees and the development of trainers. For this outside education to be effective, it must be congruent with the learner's needs of the time. Those responsible for organizing outside education need to appreciate the importance of the in-practice learning and integrate with it, recognizing the staging (Chapter 4) and the trainee's personal agenda (see Chapters 7 and 8).

SELECTION OF TRAINEES

Choosing the appropriate candidate is a problem for both the three-year scheme and the one-off situation. A substantial proportion of GP trainees in the United Kingdom are on the former and need to be selected, not only for general practice training, but also for an SHO post in a number of different specialities. This means that there could be as many as a dozen people with very differing views on the ideal candidate. It is important, therefore, that all those involved get together to define a common candidate specification and an effective method of selection. The trainers' group can provide the impetus for this development by discussing, together with the hospital consultants, the features of the ideal trainee for the scheme and agreeing a common specification.

One-off trainees can offer a scheme many advantages—variety, different perspectives, and experiences—but they can also present difficulties. The importance of trying to organize the release course with the individual staging and learning agendas of the different trainees has been touched upon (see Chapters 4 and 8), with trainees coming in at different times in the year this is very difficult. For the scheme to work effectively, the one-off trainee should start at the same time as the main entry into the scheme to allow co-ordination of the scheme and practice. The course organizer should be involved in trainee selection because a substantial part of the trainee's education will be at the release course.

THE HALF-DAY OR DAY-RELEASE COURSE

Why is there any need for out-of-practice teaching at all, and what can it offer to the trainee?

The essential advantages of this type of education are as follows:

- wider context of practice;
- encouraging conceptual thinking about practice;
- introduction of a wider range of resources;
- checking out ideas and practice with a peer group;
- developing values and attitudes;
- support and encouragement by the trainee group.

Probably the most important feature of external education is what it has to offer in terms of broadening the trainee's education and putting it into a wider context. It enables principles to be looked at and allows the issues to be discussed away from individual patients. For the trainee to develop skills and working patterns that will last for the whole of a career in general practice, the teaching must move from the specific to the general by emphasizing the principles behind the day-to-day practice.

Example:
The day-release session on health promotion was planned, with each of the trainees bringing examples of protocols from their respective practices. The group, with the help of the health promotion officer, looked at some of the broader aspects of health promotion that were missing from the programmes: the assessment of needs of specific groups, effective communication for health, and aspects of community development for health.

This is possible within the practice, but is very difficult. By centralizing extramural education, for example at the postgraduate centre, it is possible to introduce specialists from the hospital, general practice, or from outside medicine (e.g. a management consultant). The other reason that education outside the practice is essential is that it enables both the trainer and trainee to meet and discuss the issues of their work with their peers. This enables each learner to place his or her own work into the broader context of general practice. Meeting small groups also facilitates the discussion of issues that are more difficult to learn in any other settings, especially values and attitudes. Small-group learning, whether it be the trainee group on the VTS or the local trainers' group, can be very supportive and can give encouragement and enthusiasm to carry on when times are difficult. Good teaching practices can go a long way towards broadening the education for the trainee, but it must be admitted that in some places the only way a trainee can get a broader scholarly look at general practice is at the day-release course.

Although every vocational training scheme has a release course of some sort, they vary considerably from district to district. In some areas of the country, outside education for trainees consists of a series of residential courses, in others a day or half-day each week for either the 3 years or only for the GP year.

The most common format is that of a half-day-or day-release course each week for the duration of the trainee year. The same principles apply, however, to other patterns of outside practice education for trainees. The significance of the learner's agenda in adult education and the importance of personalizing the teaching to take that agenda into account have been raised earlier (see Chapters 2 and 4). It is practically impossible to personalize teaching in a large group, which is partly why most release courses use small groups. This teaching method requires specific skills from the organizers or leaders in order that the learning experience is maximized. It also means that groups of more than 12–15 trainees become increasingly difficult to manage.

PLANNING THE COURSE

Who sets the aims and objective for the course? Several people could be legitimately involved: the regional advisor, who is ultimately responsible for the scheme; the course organizer, who organizes and administers the course; the trainers, who are responsible for the majority of the trainees' teaching; and the trainees themselves.

The regional advisor, through the advisors and the course organizer group, can develop general guidelines on the structure and overall aims of the release course. An example of this would be general regional guidance that a full day per week be set aside for the release course and that every trainee is expected to attend. Another more recent example is the need to include in each release course the theoretical training for child surveillance.

The course organizer should provide the vision and the guidance for the whole scheme. He or she is often an experienced teacher with a broad view of general practice. Many course organizers take on all aspects of the job, setting aims and objectives, organizing methods, and taking a major part in the teaching.

The trainers, if properly motivated and with the appropriate knowledge and skills, are in a good position to set the aims and objectives for the course. They have close contact with their own trainees and are aware of their requirements. If they are involved in both planning and teaching, learning on the release course and in the practice can be co-ordinated and interlinked. This requires the trainers to have a clear idea of their own curriculum (see Chapter 4) and how it applies to their current trainees (see Chapter 7), and for the trainers' group with the course organizer to come to a collective plan for the release course.

Example:
The trainers and course organizer were planning practice management sessions for the release course. The trainers were aware of individual needs such as practice finance. The session was planned with each of the trainees having previously been through the accounts of their training practice, and having read an article about the subject. In the session, a practice accountant and a practice manager discussed the pros and cons of each system. Afterwards, each trainee was asked to discuss the results of the session with his or her trainer to see if any improvement could be made to the practice's accounting system.

For the trainers' group to reach a consensus careful negotiation is needed because each trainer will have different priorities and teaching styles.

We have already pointed out that the difficulties are greater if there are multiple entries into the vocational training scheme from the hospital jobs or from one-off trainees. Entry of new trainees into the release course every few months makes it difficult to create cohesion in the group, and the staging of the sessions to meet the 'maturity' of individual trainees is almost impossible.

As with individual curriculum planning, it is important to involve the learners in the planning of the day-release course. This can be difficult because of different individual wants, and changes in those wants as the year progresses. However, it should be possible to reach a general consensus.

'Playschool'

Perhaps the most upsetting thing for course organizers is to have their courses referred to by the trainers, partners, and trainees as 'playschool'. It implies something that is of little value. Why does this happen?

- The course may be seen as irrelevant to everyday practice.
- The trainees may not be adequately stretched, challenged, or involved.
- The trainers may feel that doing the job is the only real way to learn.
- The partners in the training practice may resent the time that the trainee is out of the practice and feel that it is not proper work.

As discussed in Chapter 2, effective learning happens if it is felt to be relevant to the job. If this is not the case, or if the methods used are inappropriate, the course will not have the respect of the trainer or trainee. If the trainers feel that they have a major influence on the planning and are involved in individual sessions, negative attitudes disappear.

SOME PRINCIPLES OF RELEASE-COURSE PLANNING

- The methods of setting aims of courses have been discussed, and the advantage of formulating these aims within the trainers' group (of which the course organizers are members) are stressed.
- There should be variety and change of pace throughout the day. An example of this might be three sessions in the day, with the morning

and afternoon sessions being subject based and the middle session being a case discussion or journal club.

- For each of the subject sessions a trainer and a trainee could be designated who will be responsible for organizing and running the session.
- If at all possible, the year will start at the time when most of the trainees enter the scheme, and the subject matter and teaching methods should progress throughout the year. An example of this progression is: from knowledge to skills and attitudes; from clinical subjects to organizational subjects; externally resourced learning to internally resourced learning; and from telling to self-learning.
- There should be preparation and post-session work by all the trainees for each session. This could involve, for instance, an audit or reading, discussion with team members, or a tutorial in practice.
- Each session should have written objectives beforehand and evaluations afterwards, circulated to all trainers.

Example:
The half-yearly planning in one scheme was based on the previous year's programme. It was first discussed with the trainers' group, together with the evaluations. Changes and additions were then made to the first draft programme. This was then discussed with the trainee group. They wished to add or subtract sessions, often in the first 6 months, wanted to add even more 'ear, nose, and throat' and eyes and take out the social science inputs. This trend was mainly resisted on the grounds that at this early stage there were differences between the trainees' wants and the trainees' needs. In the second half-year, when the trainees were 'practising trainees or practitioners', their suggestion for alterations to the course were welcomed.

The final programme was circulated to all trainers and trainees so that they could plan each session and arrange their in-practice learning to co-ordinate with it. Each session was evaluated by the trainees at the end of the day and forms were completed referring to the content, method, relevance, and presentation. These forms were used in planning the next year's programme.

The trainer and the release course

The trainers can be involved in the day-release course in a number of different ways that might vary from scheme to scheme and from trainer to trainer:

- planning the programme;
- within the sessions:
  observer for his/her own interest and learning;
  GP voice or opinion, to add the GP perspective to a session with another expert, e.g. gynaecologist or physiotherapist;
  organizer and co-ordinator, to plan the session, arrange any experts needed and brief them, set the objectives and the pre-session work, run the session, and plan the evaluation;
  small-group leader in the case discussion or journal club;
  expert teacher or resource, covering special interests, such as diabetic

care, practice finance, counselling, consultation video analysis, minor surgery, or psychosexual counselling.

A trainer group that feels responsible for the release course, does not describe it as 'playschool' and the trainees are more likely to attend regularly. The trainers themselves develop a confidence in their own teaching and differing expertise in a number of different fields.

RESIDENTIAL COURSES

Most trainees go on residential courses at some time during their training. These can be organized at regional or district level and may vary from introductory courses to intensive specialist courses, for example on counselling, child developmental assessment, or coping with death. Residential courses have many advantages. Trainees are together for longer periods of time without the pressures of day-to-day work. This allows the participants to develop a mutual trust that can accelerate learning and allow discussion about subjects that might never be touched on at a weekly release course (see also Chapter 2).

THE TRAINERS' GROUP

We have already referred briefly to the importance of the trainers' group in Chapter 6. Various individuals have a stake in each vocational training scheme. The trainers' priority is to organize learning for an individual trainee. Course organizers need to have a programme that has to be planned ahead for a variety of trainees. Regional advisors have to guide the content and monitor the standards. We believe that the trainers must play a major role in their scheme. They should define the candidate specification for applicants and participate in the selection of trainees for the scheme. In addition, they should maintain contact in the hospital years and provide personal tutorage. They should help define specific objectives and resource the day-release course, albeit with co-ordination and supervision from the course organizers and advisors.

This proposed increased role and responsibility of the trainers has implications for the trainers' group and its relationship with the course organizer. If the trainers' group has autonomy of decision making, then it has to take responsibility for standards of the scheme. High-quality trainers will demand and encourage high-quality day-release courses and schemes. To achieve this, the trainers will need help, guidance, education, and support from the course organizer and the regional adviser.

The majority of trainers in the country relate to, and are members of, a group of local trainers. However, these trainers' groups vary widely in their role, function, structure, and activity. They range from unstructured irregular meetings to structured assemblies with minutes and agendas, or a series of residential meetings with teaching activities. This variety often reflects geography, regional policy, or tradition, but in many cases it reflects a lack of clear ideas of the group.

Functions

It is essential that the trainers' meetings work properly. There are many different possible functions. An effective group can achieve a number of functions at once (although it is impossible to please all of the people all of the time).

Management of the scheme

In addition to the release course, other aspects need attention—selection, hospital jobs, trainees' study leave, to name but a few.

Support/problem-solving

Most trainers would agree that at times training can be a lonely and stressful job: when the trainee becomes uncommunicative; when the tutorials seem to drop like lead balloons; when the partners become resentful of the time out of the practice. At these times a group of like-minded colleagues, who have suffered similar problems, can be very helpful. They may well have ideas and possible solutions and, even if they do not, problems are often put into perspective by sharing them. These problems are often minor and self-limiting but occasionally they can be major, such as a situation involving drugs or alcohol, or where a trainer is concerned that the trainee is clinically incompetent. In these and other circumstances, the trainers' group can be the point of first contact in helping the trainer to resolve the problems. If all the trainers are involved in the release course, they can share their individual experiences of the trainees on the course with each other, offering an informed basis for that support.

Peer referencing and standard setting

By sharing ideas and experiences, trainers can check out their own proposals.

Example:
The trainers discussed assessment and the difficulties members were having with giving feedback to the trainees. John said he found it better for both trainer and trainee to fill in an assessment from on each other and then share the results of both assessments. Diana, a new trainer, looked relieved, as she confessed that this was the method she used but felt guilty because it was not the 'correct way'. Several of the trainers felt more relaxed about assessment at the end of the discussion.

Support from a group of trainers doing the same job and wishing to help each other improve is a most effective way of raising the standard of training locally. If one of the members of the group does not measure up, the subtle pressure from the others in a supportive atmosphere helps things to change.

Trainer development

The trainers' group can be a very effective vehicle for trainer development. Courses and reading can stimulate ideas, but often those ideas are lost if it is not possible to practise them in a supportive atmosphere. Examples of trainers' groups arranging the professional development of their members are:

- Some look at their videotaped consultations and/or tutorials together and give each other feedback.
- Some will arrange outside assistance, such as an adult educationalist, a management consultant, or another GP with a special interest.
- Some set themselves a project to research and develop, e.g. a joint training log; an assessment package; a selection technique.
- Some develop a scheme trainee assessment, with the trainers visiting and assessing the trainee and training, and then giving feedback to the trainer and trainee.
- Some carry out a joint clinical audit that involves all the training practices, and publish the results.
- Some develop their small-group leadership skills with the help of a facilitator.
- Some set up exchanges with trainers and trainees in other regions and countries. Various other initiatives could be undertaken, depending on local circumstances and needs.

Structure and process

Any group of people, unless a purely social gathering, needs to get the correct balance of tasks that need to be achieved and activities that maintain the cohesion of the group. Some aspects should be considered:

Size

It is very difficult for a group larger than 12–15 people to take in the needs of each of the members. In larger towns and cities the trainer groups often divide into smaller units.

Dividing the group

The splitting of the group can produce problems with the process of the whole group and there has to be a continual review of the needs of all the members and the balance between the task in hand and the process of the group.

Frequency and length of meetings

However well people know each other, it takes many minutes for them to re-establish contact when meeting anew. With the tendency of GPs to be late and a need to leave early, 1–2 hours at lunchtime is often spent mainly with hellos and goodbyes. Many trainer groups meet once a month at lunchtime, and become frustrated because nothing ever happens. Probably the effective pattern is to meet less often for longer periods of time. This provides members with the time for reflection that is lacking in everyday practice.

Shared aims for the group meeting

It can be very frustrating for the group members if everyone has a different perception as to why he or she is there. Planned agendas and brief minutes or action plans can help.

Practical working using real examples

One of the most powerful tools of the trainers' group in developing the teaching professionalism of its members is the use of video-recordings of consultations or tutorials. Other techniques can also contribute to this process, e.g. role play, case discussion, using and sharing teaching tools, etc.

Initiation of new members

New or potential trainers can find entering a long-running group difficult. Language, code of behaviour, and rituals are already established. The course organizer or group chairman needs to be aware of this, and to have a system of introduction. Many schemes appoint a more experienced trainer as a mentor or supporter to aid this difficult transition.

Problems with individual trainers

Individuals within the group can often behave in a very disruptive manner. They can be aggressive; exclusive of others; intransigent; superior; or non-participating. The reasons for this inappropriate behaviour are manifold but often have their basis in other spheres of life. If a trainer comes to the meeting angry at a partner, or anxious about a family matter, his or her behaviour at the meeting may reflect these problems. Some trainers can block development of the group from time to time, producing intense frustration in other members.

THE COURSE OR VOCATIONAL TRAINING SCHEME ORGANIZER

Leading a group of independent-minded GP trainers and trainees is a difficult task which is usually undertaken by the course organizer. The leader must be aware of the range of individual behaviour within the group and able to act accordingly. He or she needs a range of skills: group leadership, administration, and teaching.

This chapter has dwelt on the importance of the close working relationship between the course organizer and the trainers in the development of release courses. This relationship is equally important in all the other aspects of the scheme—the hospital jobs, selection, the trainer group, etc. The course organizer is in a position to provide leadership to the scheme, to give vision and inspiration to all the members of the scheme, and help them all in their development.

The course organizer is often in a difficult position, having to relate to the regional advisor on one hand and the trainers' group on the other. It is important, therefore, that he or she has the support of both these parties and is able to exercise appropriate leadership

THE REGIONAL AND ASSOCIATE ADVISORS

The regional advisors are responsible to the post graduate dean for the vocational training of general practitioners, and how that responsibility is interpreted varies from region to region. In some cases central control remains, maintained by regional advisors and associates, while in others the responsibility is developed to the course organizers and trainers' groups.

Trainer selection and reselection is the responsibility of the regional GP educational committe; how this actually happens varies from region to region. Throughout this book, with the principles of adult learning and the development of trainee responsibility, we have emphasized the importance of individuals feeling responsible for their own educational development. This principle applies to training practices also. The setting and monitoring of standards of training practices ideally should be a peer-group activity, with all the trainers being involved, as at Oxford (Schofield and Hasler 1984). This makes each assessment visit an educational activity for both the visited and the visitors (see Chapter 11).

Probably the most important function of the region is the educational development of the course organizers and the trainers. Regional training courses play a major part in setting the standards and helping people reach them. These training courses can be standard teaching courses or special-interest courses involved in the teaching of communication or management skills. Many regional advisers also set up study days to encourage the exchange of ideas throughout the region.

Regional advisers have to learn how to exercise leadership, involving all those concerned in vocational training while presenting a clear vision for the future. A region develops its identity in the balance between control and support, between helping and telling, and between freedom and monitoring. If one wishes to help trainees develop into independent self-sufficient individuals, the whole administrative structure must reflect that ethos.

National representation and contacts

It is very important that a region maintains contact with others. The advisor structure both formally and informally encourages this. The cosmopolitan outlook can be extended to interregional course organizer and trainer meetings.

In this chapter, understandably, we have concentrated on the VTS when considering outside-practice teaching and support, but the chapter would not be complete without considering the postgraduate centre.

POST GRADUATE CENTRE

Postgraduate centres are changing. Seen originally as largely a building with a lecture theatre, seminar rooms, and libraries with stocks of books, they are now being seen as important resource centres for the whole district.

Most VTS release courses are run in the postgraduate centre, are administered by the centre administrator, and the centre is central to the whole scheme. It is important that the trainees are aware of, and benefit from, the other activities of the centre. A major activity is the continuing medical education (CME) programme for GP principals. Sharing of resources, liaison on study days, and co-operation with programmes makes obvious sense. The re-emergence of medical audit with the new contract, requires the introduction of quality measurement and assurance to the trainees and certainly to the trainers' practices.

Trainees need to know how to use library facilities. This involves not merely having access to an up-to-date range of textbooks, including ones on general practice, but also being familiar with how to carry out literature searches and use appropriate information technology. The librarian is an important resource.

CONCLUSIONS

The importance of resources outside the training practice has been stressed. In particular:

- Trainee selection needs to be done professionally.

- *Release courses must be planned to complement practice teaching and involve the trainers. The entry of scheme and one-off trainees should be co-ordinated with the start of each course, which should mirror the staging process of the trainee year.
- Trainers should accept some of the responsibility for making their trainers' group function. Course organizers need good small-group leadership skills and should be aware of factors that help or hinder the group.
- Postgraduate centre resources should be exploited to the full.
- Regional advisers should provide vision while involving course organizers and trainers in their own development.

10 Learning in hospital

Most of this book is concerned with training in general practice but this is only one part of the 3 years of preparation for general practice. A wide range of experiences has been reported by doctors in hospital training grades. A number of posts have broad-based educational programmes, learning objectives, protected time set aside, and the involvement of SHOs in their own learning. Unfortunately this is not the experience of many SHOs; whether or not their career goal is general practice. All junior hospital posts are training posts requiring time and expertise for planned learning. In this chapter we examine three issues—the balance between education and service, the function of SHO posts, and the purpose of hospital training for GPs—and then go on to consider various aspects of the posts.

Some of the issues raised concern the whole structure of medical education; these are also discussed in Part 3. A particular example of such an issue is the amount of training in general practice as opposed to hospital posts. Concern has been expressed about the balance between the hospital and general practice components of training for future general practitioners (Byrne 1975). In particular, it seems anomalous that two-thirds of vocational training should be spent in a hospital environment. We shall argue for a greater amount of time to be spent in practice, but that this should not be at the expense of training in hospital. We wish to stress the important role that hospital posts and specialists have in the training of future general practitioners. The learning of many skills which are best acquired in hospital are essential to the development of doctors who will work in primary care. It is important, therefore, that the range of experience is appropriate to the needs of the trainee's future career. Equally, we believe that there must be a considerable service commitment in posts. Indeed, this is part of the value of the experience.

CURRENT ISSUES

Balance between education and service

It has long been accepted that there is an imbalance between service commitment and education (Council for Postgraduate Medical Education in England and Wales 1987). The transfer of the budget for part of each SHO post to deans should allow a proper emphasis on education (National Health Service Management Executive 1991). However, postgraduate deans and advisers in general practice will need to exert their authority in order to ensure proper experiences for all training grades, including general practitioner vocational trainees in SHO posts.

There is little disagreement about the desirability of improving the educational opportunities in all SHO posts: in particular, there is a great willingness to increase the amount of teaching. The pressures on senior staff have never been greater, however, and managers have to be persuaded of the necessity of affording training a high priority. It is not clear what effect the expansion of trust status will have in this area. The identification of an educational budget which is the responsibility of postgraduate deans offers a way of ensuring that the appropriate priority is accorded to teaching and learning, but mechanisms must be put into place rapidly to secure this.

If a training post is to yield its full potential, it must encourage the trainee to make the most of the experience. Part of this is to ensure the correct balance between service and education. However, trainees will not be able to reflect on their experiences, experiment with different methods, and carry out projects or other exercises if they are too tired or if the pressure of work simply does not allow sufficient time. Much anecdotal evidence suggests that exhaustion lies at the base of the loss of motivation experienced by junior doctors. This is exacerbated by the dissatisfaction felt as a result of carrying out important and very sensitive tasks in a rushed and impersonal way. The working considerations must therefore provide time and appropriate surroundings for effective working, relaxation, and study.

While there has been some improvement as a result of recent government initiatives, our experience with SHOs in the hard-pressed specialities suggests that a very high proportion are still working between 64 and 73 hours a week. The difficulties of making the SHO post truly educational are many, particularly with the staffing and on-call requirements that are now needed.

At the present time debate continues as to whether SHO posts are generic—that is, providing a common pathway for all specialities including general practice, or whether they should differ according to the ultimate goals of the trainees.

Many of the needs of doctors in hospital posts are clearly similar to those of GP trainees. The differences between the needs of GP trainees and those of doctors following careers in hospital medicine at the SHO grade have been, and remain, matters of debate. On the one hand, it may be that the required skills may differ, but much of the knowledge and many of the skills and attitudes are common to both. The maintenance of a distinction may result in the maximum benefit being obtained, but separation exacts a price. The price is partly organizational and partly attitudinal, with GP trainees expecting, and receiving, different treatment. This may exclude them from the team and result in isolation which is unhelpful to individuals and harmful to the development of a common approach to education.

The General Medical Council has constructed a list of aims of training for doctors (General Medical Council 1987). These aims recognize a much wider agenda than that usually perceived for junior hospital staff. The areas covered are:

1. The ability to solve clinical and other problems in medical practice.
2. Possession of adequate knowledge and understanding of the general structure and function of the human body and workings of the mind, in health and disease, of their interaction between man and his physical and social environments.
3. Possession of consultation skills.
4. Acquisition of a high standard of knowledge and skills in the doctor's specialty.
5. Willingness and ability to deal with common medical emergencies and with other illnesses in an emergency.
6. The ability to contribute appropriately to the prevention of illness and the promotion of health.
7. The ability to recognize and analyse ethical problems so as to enable patients, their family, society, and the doctor to have a proper regard to such problems in reaching decisions.
8. The maintenance of attitudes and conduct appropriate to a high level of professional practice.
9. Mastery of the skills required to work within a team and, where appropriate, assume the responsibilities of team leader.
10. Acquisition of experience in administration and planning.
11. Recognition of the opportunities and acceptance of the duty to contribute, when possible, to the advancement of medical knowledge and skill.
12. Recognition of the obligation to teach others, particularly doctors in training.

The General Medical Council included more details under each of these headings, which make even clearer the relevance to training for general practice. It seems, therefore, that there would be great advantage in identifying the hospital experience as a period of general professional training to be followed by specialist training, which in the case of general practitioners would take place in general practice. A potential disadvantage of this would be the loss of specifically relevant learning experiences. These might be better exploited by a system of training in which the hospital component is an important but subsidiary part of an overall plan of preparation for work in primary care.

The function of hospital training for general practitioners

If hospital training is to be a part of specialist training for general practice, rather than general professional training, its purpose has to be explored in a different light. In particular, there may be a problem about the relevance of some aspects of posts. An obvious example is provided by neonatology in paediatric work. It may be useful for trainees to have some experience of specialized tasks in order to know what is involved, both from the technical point of view and from the viewpoint of patients experiencing care. However, the main thrust should be towards the acquisition of important skills in the management of more common situations. Individual posts therefore need to be examined with these issues in mind. A format for discussion of individual posts has been provided by the RCGP, working with a number of other Royal Colleges and organizations, which should help to focus on appropriate learning objectives (Royal College of General Practitioners 1993). See also Appendix VI.

ASPECTS OF SHO POSTS

Whatever developments occur in the future, the issue of effectiveness in teaching and learning needs to be addressed as a matter of urgency, and there are several other important areas to be resolved. These may be considered under the following headings:

- effective teaching and learning;
- working conditions;
- GP participation and relationship with schemes;
- release courses;
- study leave;
- selection and recruitment;
- development and maintenance of standards;
- problems of one-off trainees.

Effective teaching and learning

Problems have been perceived with both the objectives of learning in hospital posts and in the way that training takes place (Reeve and Bowman 1989; Kearly 1990). The adoption and mutual agreement of objectives, selection of appropriate methods, and the use of valid and reliable assessment tools together form the educational cycle whose principles have been the main subjects of this book. Many of the concerns that have been explored in relation to teaching and learning in general practice apply equally to hospital posts. However, their application in the hospital setting is largely a matter for consultant and middle-grade staff. GP trainers and course organizers may be able to assist in this process by sharing their own experiences and joint learning exercises. Attempts at dictating teaching methods deny the principles of adult learning, and risk losing both goodwill and valuable expertise.

Several initiatives are aimed at developing teaching skills in hospital posts, which have been the subject of recent studies (SCOPME; Coles *et al.* 1993) and also work in the Kettering and Windsor districts within our own region.

Formal contracts should include the educational as well as other aspects of training posts. At the same time, trainees and their educational supervisors, whether in hospital or GP, should be encouraged to agree informal learning contracts which reflect their particular needs and include objectives, methods, and assessment.

The utility and value of training logs have been discussed in Chapter 7. Such records are as applicable in hospital posts as they are in general practice. The widespread use of such records by all SHOs who may enter general practice, or possibly by all doctors in the grade, would focus attention on the educational aspects of their work and encourage some continuity of education. Even where posts are not linked to schemes, or are undertaken by doctors whose future careers are uncertain, it is important that they still have educational objectives and that training and assessment are well documented, so that experiences have the maximum effect wherever the doctor goes subsequently.

Time must be recognized as a major issue. Although we have urged that due recognition be given to education alongside service, there will never be sufficient time to meet all the possible objectives of SHO posts. Therefore techniques will need to be developed to make the best use of these posts, including the maximum use of administrative and clinical support for SHOs and the development of strategies to obtain the maximum learning from limited opportunities. An example of such strategies is given by the 'bench packages' developed for learning in short periods of time between tasks (Grant *et al.* 1989).

People in training also need feedback on the progress that they are making in their work. This should be related to more formal educational assessment, but at least some appraisal of their work is needed both for reassurance and development. This must be sufficiently explicit for all to know that it is occurring, although there are varying degrees of formality. It also needs to allow the trainee to make suggestions for improvement in the post, so the appraisal is mutual.

Working conditions

We have referred to the need to reduce the pressure on junior doctors and to avoid the dissatisfaction resulting from excessive hours and pressure. However, there is also a need to ensure that living conditions, including accommodation and catering arrangements, are satisfactory. These are often grossly inadequate in hospitals and the result is demoralization.

Earlier generations of doctors felt that they were valued when they were working as juniors, even though the working conditions were often grossly inadequate. The value put on them was manifest by specific arrangements for catering and a clear effort on the part of authorities to ensure that junior doctors were well treated. This sense of being valued appears not to exist any longer in some hospitals. Although we recognize that this change is part of many others affecting a range of professions, specific measures are needed to support staff working under what may at times be intolerable pressure.

GP participation and relationship with schemes

Although training in hospital may be largely the concern of senior hospital staff, there are broadly two ways in which general practitioners may work with hospital staff in relation to SHO posts. The generalist perspective is important for the purpose of general professional training, and general practitioners have important insights to offer to the education of all SHOs. If the initial SHO posts become part of a clearly defined general professional training, the GP input will be more easily identified. However, even with the present arrangements, general practitioners have much to offer the training of junior staff in hospitals.

In addition, GP trainers are able to offer specific inputs into the training of junior staff whose final career path is general practice. Many SHO posts are linked to vocational training rotations and, in these cases, trainees benefit from seeing the hospital experience as part of a coherent programme. This may include agreement between the hospital and GP authorities as to the contribution of each. Reference has already been made to the series of documents produced by the Royal College of General Practitioners with other Royal College setting out the objectives of training in a number of clinical areas, which are intended to provide bases for such local discussions (Royal College of General Practitioners 1993).

Teaching during hospital posts may involve GP trainers who may be able to offer a different perspective on hospital experiences which are of benefit to all. This is in keeping with the concept of SHO posts being regarded as general professional training. In some schemes it has been helpful to have GPs who act as links between schemes and individual departments (Oxford Region Course Organisers and Advisors Group 1988).

Release courses

Another way in which trainees may keep in touch with their chosen career path is through day, or more commonly half-day, release. There is always a debate about the relationship between the release course and SHO posts. In some schemes, trainees are able to attend a course throughout the whole of their 3 year period of training. In others, those in hospital posts are excluded completely, while in many schemes the situation is variable or confused.

It is difficult to make the 3 year schemes truly 3 years of co-ordinated education towards general practice, rather than the 2 years in hospital and 1 year in practice seen at present in the majority. The problems lie both with the SHOs, who feel they are obstetricians when they are doing obstetrics and psychiatrists when they are psychiatry SHOs, and with the consultants, who often lose sight of the chosen career of their SHOs. Unfortunately, there are difficulties in some hospitals where the SHOs are regarded as being there to provide a service, their learning needs often seen as secondary; a problem that is no different for career specialist SHOs or those on the VTS. With the increasing problems that consultants have with management and budgeting on top of their clinical responsibilities, teaching can often be a low priority. This was demonstrated by findings presented to the 1990 National Trainee Conference and further confirmed the authors' own experiences of visiting SHO posts in the Oxford region (Crawley and Levin 1990).

Several issues should be considered, of which the most important is educational. Most authorities on general practice have urged attendance by trainees throughout a 3 year course, pointing to the need for continuing support from colleagues, the maintenance of the general practice perspective, and the greater range of topics that can be covered. Conversely, it may be difficult for trainees to get much benefit from discussions on topics that are unrelated to the posts they are filling at the time. The other main issue is usually a logistic one. Problems are posed to many hospital departments by the regular absence of SHOs at fixed times, and this is a particular difficulty in relatively small units and hospitals. There may also be a problem of attitudes; some hospital departments are unsympathetic to the attendance of SHOs at GP release schemes. Equally, some trainees do not wish to be regarded differently from their hospital colleagues and resent pressure on them to attend.

The options available to those with responsibility for training SHOs include:

• provision of common educational programmes for all SHOs;
• release of GP trainees to separate release courses;
• the attendance of GP trainees at special courses outside the hospital programme.

It is unlikely that a single solution will be appropriate for all situations, but it should not be acceptable for junior doctors in training grades to forego regular formal education. Also, GP trainees should not be put in the position of having training at the expense of their hospital colleagues. If education is to be provided separately, both groups should have appropriate programmes. However, there does seem to be a case for flexibility in the demands of organizers of vocational training schemes. There may be advantages in encouraging trainees to take part in the educational programme of their present post, provided that there are other mechanisms for continuing the links with vocational training. Such mechanisms may include additional meetings run by the local VTS, regular release to training practices or more formal courses, perhaps three times a year as is currently arranged in the south-western region (Gray, personal communication 1994).

Study leave

Where a significant amount of time is spent on GP educational programmes, it may be appropriate for these to use up part of the entitlement to study leave. Indeed, this may be the only basis on which such an arrangement can be made. However, there should still be some entitlement to study leave for specific purposes. It is important that study leave can be granted for activities that do not necessarily relate to the current post being filled by the trainee if the study will benefit his or her ultimate career.

Selection and recruitment

We referred to this in Chapter 9. The responsibility for the recruitment and selection of trainees is usually divided between a number of people working both in general practice and in hospitals. This joint decision making may be a strength, but the division of responsibility may lead to a lack of clear objectives. A mixture of agendas exists, including those of hospital departments, personnel departments, practices, trainee groups, and the future of general practice. These differing interests are usually served without conflict, but this is not always the case, and it is the responsibility of schemes to ensure that decision making is explicit, with criteria that safeguard entry into primary care. Special difficulties may be created if there is a general reduction in the standard of applicants for places in training, and these should be met by refusal to compromise.

Development and maintenance of standards

The development of standards of education in SHO posts will need encouragement and a supporting framework. The current system of Royal College visits has had some influence in building up the infrastructure of training posts, protecting staffing levels, but it does not occur with sufficient frequency or allow enough time to look at educational methods in detail. We have found that this task can, however, be performed successfully by a visiting network involving the postgraduate dean, advisers in general practice, and specialty advisers. The main purpose of such a network is to encourage development, but it is also a process of accreditation and reaccreditation, so minimum standards can be maintained at the same time.

CONCLUSIONS

Several issues have to be addressed on a national scale, and some of these are examined in Part 3 of this book. Of more immediate relevance to those working in general practice and hospitals how is the question of how to help make the hospital jobs better from an educational point of view and more relevant to GP trainees holding the posts. The basis of this development is closer contact and co-operation between general practitioners and consultants in vocational training schemes, to overcome the lack of mutual trust and respect that is so often encountered. The solutions to these problems have to be pursued on at least two fronts: enhancing education for all junior doctors and encouraging greater contact within vocational training schemes.

In order to enhance the education of all junior doctors there is a need to:

- adopt agreed objectives, appropriate methods, and valid assessment for all trainees;
- establish visiting of SHO posts by mixed GP/specialist teams to look at and approve the standards of education in the departments;
- establish joint trainer/consultant working groups in subject areas;
- develop joint learning between hospital doctors and general practitioners in subjects related to education, such as presentation skills, interviewing skills, assessment, and curriculum planning

Measures to encourage greater contacts within vocational schemes include:

- mutual assessment of posts and trainees by GP trainers, course organizers, and consultants, allowing feedback of the experience within SHO posts;
- involving consultants in discussions and teaching on the release course, enabling them to appreciate the problems of general practice as it relates to their speciality;
- continuing personal tutorage of the GP trainees in SHO posts by GP trainers;
- involving trainees in general practice more formally, during or before their hospital jobs. An introductory 1 or 2 months before the SHO jobs followed by 10 or 11 months afterwards is a common pattern.

Appendix VI sets out the Oxford criteria for education in junior hospital posts.

11 Evaluating the teaching

In his review of training for general practice, published in 1982, Pereira Gray asked the question 'Does vocational training work?' and concluded, on the basis of available evidence, that no study satisfactorily demonstrated that vocationally trained general practitioners provided a better standard of care than untrained practitioners. The same remains true today, and indeed some evidence, such as that of Cartwright and Anderson (1981), indicates that there was no significant difference between trained and untrained general practitioners in the way they viewed their patients or the satisfaction they obtained from their work.

This situation is understandable. The only satisfactory evidence would have been obtained from a controlled trial. In the early days vocational training was only undertaken by volunteers who were not comparable with those who entered general practice directly, and after 1981 vocational training was mandatory for all doctors.

In this chapter we examine the purpose of evaluation and the questions it can answer, identify what can be evaluated, and then go on to examine various approaches and what can be done in practice.

THE PURPOSE OF EVALUATION

The most valuable purpose of evaluation is to determine the effectiveness of an individual session or an educational programme at achieving its objectives, in order that it may be maintained and improved in the future. It should therefore be an integral part of the organization of education, and all teachers should be involved in the continued evaluation of their own work. The information that evaluation provides can also be used to enhance the quality of the debate about the development of good practice in education.

In addition, evaluation can be used to explore other issues, such as value for money and the relationship of the education to external criteria, to decide whether the educational programme or teacher should continue. Evaluation can explore more difficult questions, such as what the value system is underpinning the education, who is setting the criteria, and whose interests are being served by them. In other words, why is teaching conducted in any particular way?

Evaluation can be internal, conducted by those who are responsible for the education, or it can be external; but in both cases it is essential to establish the preconceptions of the evaluators, the purpose of the evaluation, and whose interests are being served.

It is helpful to draw the distinction between 'assessment', which is based on the competence of the learner, and 'evaluation', which is based on the effectiveness of the teacher. What they have in common is that both can either be formative, leading to change and development, or summative, leading to decisions about accreditation and approval (see Chapter 5).

QUESTIONS THAT EVALUATION CAN ANSWER

Evaluation needs to have clearly formulated questions to answer, even if the information available is only subjective.

What actually happens during the tutorial, training session, or vocational training programme?

As a first step it is necessary to describe what actually happens in as objective a manner as possible. This observation needs to be open and wide-ranging, and the evaluation needs to take account of the perspectives of all those involved in the education. The evaluators must be rigorous about their own preconceptions and the basis on which any judgements are made.

What goals have been set for the teaching, who set them, and are they appropriate?

These goals may be stated explicitly, or the teacher may be making implicit assumptions that need to be explored. There may also be external or political factors that are helping shape what is provided. Appropriateness needs to be judged in relation to the needs of the learners, and to the needs of any other agencies or groups whose interests should be served, for example in the context of vocational training, the trainee's future patients. On the other hand, the training may be organized to meet the needs of the funders, and education may have to take second place to service provision.

Is the education meeting these goals?

One problem is that the question 'Does vocational training work?' is too global in its scope and too difficult to answers particularly in the absence of generally agreed measures of good-quality care. It is much easier to consider each component of training separately and to set goals to be achieved in that component. It is also more valuable, as the information obtained can be used to inform change in that component of the training.

How can the teaching and learning be improved?

This is the fundamental question that the evaluators should be asking. The answer depends on being able to identify the components of the teaching that contribute to its effectiveness and therefore need to be preserved and developed, as well as those that need to be changed. For example, a global rating of small-group teaching on the day-release course may indicate dissatisfaction, but fuller enquiry may discover that the timing of the sessions and the variable membership of the group are the causes of the difficulties, whereas the group leader is valued highly.

A final question, which has been asked rarely in the past but will undoubtably become more salient in the future, is 'Is this teaching good value for money?' This involves looking critically not only at the direct costs of providing the training, but also at the indirect and opportunity costs of this activity compared to other ways that the time and resources could be used.

WHAT CAN BE EVALUATED?

The structure–process–outcome model proposed by Donabedian (1966) for the assessment of medical care is equally applicable to the evaluation of education.

Structural aspects include such things as the context in which the training takes place, the facilities and resources in training practices, the selection process for trainees, the training of teachers, the involvement of trainers in the design of day-release courses, and the framework for assessment and accreditation of trainees.

The process of the teaching and learning is what actually takes place between teacher and learner, and between the learner and the content of the learning. This covers such issues as the way the agenda is set, the appropriateness of teaching methods, and the relationship between learner and teacher. It is very important to establish that the elements of process that are examined are those that can be related to the outcomes of the teaching.

Outcomes must be defined in terms of changes in the knowledge, skills, and attitudes of the learner, which may or may not have been defined clearly as educational objectives beforehand.

For instance, in an evaluation of the effectiveness of the education provided in the practice about the organization of diabetic care, the aspects that could be considered are:

- Structure
  Presence of a clinic in the training practice and its accessibility to the trainee.
  The involvement of the practice nurse in teaching.
  The quality of the medical records and practice register.
  The literature available in the practice library.
- Process

Is the teaching planned so that the trainee learns about basic diabetic care early in the year, and methods of setting up a clinic towards the end? (See Chapter 4.)

If there is to be a tutorial on this topic, are the trainee's questions and needs clearly defined and met?

Are the trainees encouraged to define problems in this area and to find their own solutions to them?

What use is made of the training opportunities of feedback from diabetic patients?

How much time has a trainee spent in seeing patients, attending the clinic, and leaning about diabeties?

Could this time have been spent more productively in other ways?

How much involvement has there been of partners, practice nurses, and other staff in the teaching?

- Outcomes
Is the trainee able to understand the principles involved in diabetic care?
Can the trainee manage diabetic patients in the setting of general practice?
Will the trainee be able to meet the needs of those patients?
Will the trainee be able to set up and manage a diabetic clinic in his or her own practice?

APPROACHES TO EVALUATION

Illuminative evaluation

Answering the questions 'What is happening and why?' requires a much more open approach than seeking to establish whether this teaching meets set criteria and achieves defined goals.

An open enquiry that recognizes its preconceptions but is willing and able to change them in the course of the enquiry, and is able to use a flexible range of methods to collect information, has other advantages. It acknowledges that the evaluator or teacher is not the only source of information or insight, and, by involving teachers and learners in the evaluation, increases their commitment to its outcome. The evaluator can also negotiate the questions that different parties would like answered, and provide information that contributes to the continued development of the teaching.

Multi-source evaluation

Information coming from a number of sources provides the opportunity for a process of 'triangulation', where these different observations can be used to build up a more complete picture of the effectiveness of a particular training session or programme. For example, the effectiveness of the day-release course could be evaluated from a combination of the course organizer's observations of the activity in each session, the trainees' reports on the relevance and value of each session, the views of the trainers in the trainers' group about the ideas and stimulation that the trainees bring back to the practices, and the observations of a neighbouring course organizer invited to review one day of the course.

Criterion-based evaluation

This approach depends on selecting criteria that are valid and can be assessed reliably. In other words, that the elements of structure and process are demonstrably related to outcomes and that these outcomes are desirable. To use the vexed example of training practice records, it is of little value to state that 'Training practices should have good records' without first obtaining evidence that connects summarized records with effective learning, or even effective clinical practice. Failure to do this has brought some external evaluation into disrepute. Even if the validity of a criterion is accepted, it is necessary to agree a bench-mark for its assessment, for example '80 per cent of all records should contain an up-to-date summary': it then becomes possible for the trainers themselves to evaluate whether this has been achieved.

Learner reports

The same rigour needs to be applied to the question of learner satisfaction as a indicator of educational effectiveness. Aiming to provide learner-centred teaching, or recognizing the learner as a crucially important source of information about what takes place, is not the same as regarding happy consumers as the major desirable outcome of a course. Many post-course questionnaires depend on this latter assumption, and the effect created by a warm afterglow can influence the perceptions of both learners and teachers.

Controlled experiments

Evaluating the structure and the process of teaching is very much easier than evaluating its outcome, because of the fundamental difficulty of attributing any change in the learners' abilities to their training rather than to their previous education, their normal maturation, and other external factors. The most satisfactory way is the controlled trial. This involves offering any new teaching innovation to a 'treated' group and comparing them with a 'control group' who only differ in that they have not received this particular educational experience. This needs to be done before the innovation becomes standard practice.

This is the accepted gold standard for evaluation in the clinical setting, but there are extremely few examples of this approach being taken in medical education or vocational training in the United Kingdom. This is explained partly by the difficulty in setting up the controlled experiment, and in generalizing from the experimental setting to normal practice.

EVALUATION IN PRACTICE

Evaluation of courses

Courses both for trainees and for trainers evolve in response to external factors, such as the need for new developments in practice, and in the light of the experience of those running previous courses. Systematic feedback from the course members, either using discussion sessions or questionnaires, can inform this process, but inviting an external evaluator to observe, to discuss with teachers and learners, and to take a critical and constructive look at the whole process of the course can provide a totally fresh perspective and contribute to the planning of future courses. These evaluations can be equally rigorous and more illuminating than more structured studies, but are less likely to be published in the medical literature.

The most common form of evaluation used in vocational training is the questionnaire administered at the end of a session or course. At first sight this is straightforward, but very often the questionnaires do not yield the information that the teacher requires to identify what needs to be changed in future sessions.

Open questions such as 'What did you learn from this session today?', or 'How could this course be improved?' can provoke a wide variety of views and ideas, but may be difficult to analyse and compare with other responses. Focusing the open questions may go some way towards overcoming this difficulty, for example, trainees may be invited to:

(1) list five things that they most appreciated about their training practice;
(2) list five things that they would most like to change about their training practice.

Rating scales, on the other hand, produce a numerical result which is easier to aggregate and to compare.

Example:
Please rate this session for:

	Lowest				Highest
Content	1	2	3	4	5
Presentation	1	2	3	4	5

To what extent do you agree with these statements:

	Do not agree				Strongly agree
The session was well organized	1	2	3	4	5
My interest was maintained throughout the session	1	2	3	4	5

The problem with interpreting these responses is that they do not identify areas for improvement, and the only response to low ratings may be to drop the session.

There are many examples of well-constructed questionnaires that combine open and closed questions, for example the evaluation pack produced by the Joint Centre for Education in Medicine.

Another approach developed in the Oxford Region is to ask all trainees at the end of their training to rate on a ten-point scale:

(1) the objectives for training for:
    (a)   importance, and
    (b)   achievement; and
(2) the methods used in training for:
    (a)   potential value, and
    (b)   actual value.

While the rating by each trainee depends on individual factors, the aggregated data give valuable information. For example, there is a high level of agreement about the importance of the objectives, but those relating to practice management and new technology are rated as least well achieved. Clinically based teaching methods are rated highly for potential and actual value, while those based on team activities, projects, and audit have been seen as increasingly valuable over the 8 years of data collection. It has also been possible to correlate different teaching methods with achievement of different objectives.

Tutorial evaluation

Using the task list set out in Chapter 3, it is possible to analyse a tutorial. The easiest way is to watch a videotape of the tutorial and for the trainer and trainee to assess together to what extent each task has been achieved. Although not all the tasks are always relevant, many of them are, and our experience is that the procedure is a useful way of highlighting strengths and weaknesses.

Training practice evaluation

The methodology for assessing the performance of doctors in their own practices was originally designed by a working party of the RCGP and described in its report *what sort of doctor?* (1985). The report identified four areas that could be assessed: professional values, communication, accessibility, and clinical competence. The approach has since been developed and used at Oxford for many years for assessing training practices and the training they provide (Schofield and Hasler 1984).

Applying this methodology to training practices involved the production, by a working group of trainers, of an agreed set of criteria against which they were willing to be assessed by their peers.

The method of assessment is based on a visit to the doctor's own practice by two colleagues for the better part of a day. The assessment has six components:

1. study of the practice profile, recording the salient features of the practice, circulated to the assessors in advance of the visit;
2. direct observation of the practice premises, its facilities and equipment, and the way it functions;
3. discussion with administrative staff and other members of the practice's health-care team;
4. inspection of individual clinical records and any registers or indexes the practice possesses;
5. review of a videotape of a tutorial and a series of the doctor's recent consultations, together with the relevant records;
6. an interview with the doctor to elicit his or her views and understanding on a variety of topics, including material derived from randomly selected patients' records.

Advantages of this method are that the assessment is based on direct observation of the doctor's performance in practice, and that each method of assessment provides information from which performance in a number of areas can be assessed.

At the end of the visit the visitors produce a written report summarizing the strengths and weaknesses that they have identified in each of the four areas of performance. The more the comments are specifically related to the criteria and based on specific information gained during the visit, and the more that these observations are coupled to specific recommendations for change, the greater the value of the report to the doctor and to the practice that is being visited. These reports are then considered by the trainers' appointments committee, which has the responsibility for approvals (coupled with recommendations for change or development).

Based on the experience of vocational training schemes over the past 10 years, it is possible to describe several essential requirements that ensure that assessment visiting is both acceptable to trainers and valuable in promoting the development of training practices (Schofield and Hasler 1984):

The criteria used for the assessment should be based on the consumers' needs

In the case of the training practices, the following statement of principle was made: 'Teaching practices and trainers are selected for the education opportunities they offer their trainees. Since trainees may learn from the experience and example of working in the practices well as from teaching and other educational resources, all these areas must be examined.'

The criteria must be agreed by those who are to be assessed

This may involve a fairly lengthy period of consultation with trainers and trainers' groups, but the criteria produced are more likely to be both realistic and acceptable.

The criteria must be realistic and acceptable levels of performance must be defined in relation to local circumstances

At one extreme one must avoid setting unattainable ideals and, at the other, failing to meet the responsibilities to the consumer, in this case the trainee, by making too much allowance for the problems of the practice.

All practitioners should be involved as assessors

This gives all practitioners the opportunity to learn from visiting each others' practices, but, more importantly, creates a sense of involvement in the whole process. It avoids a 'them and us' feeling and is another safeguard to ensure that the judgements that are made are realistic.

Assessors must receive training

Teams of two or three general practitioners are led by an experienced visitor who has the responsibility for conducting the visit and writing the report. Team leaders attend regular study days at which consistent problems are identified and discussed.

The report should be based on informed judgements against the agreed criteria

The report should make clear what information has been gathered in the practice and the degree to which individual criteria have or have not been met. General statements such as 'The practice has a nice atmosphere' are far less valuable than noting that 'The practice has regular meetings and all members of staff are able to add items to the agenda and feel able to express their ideas freely.' Another dimension of experience is to be able to make recommendations based not just on one's own practice but also on ideas from other practices that have been visited.

The ethos of the assessment should be to encourage development

The purpose of assessment visiting should be to develop the teaching and experience that the practice provides. The final report of the process should identify areas in which the practice should be encouraged to develop, and practices should expect to improve levels of performance between one evaluation and the next. It is also possible over time for the criteria and the acceptable levels of performance to be raised as the overall standard of the practice develops.

Resources should be available to encourage practice and trainer development

There is little point in identifying the areas of weakness if the means of improving them are not available. In the context of training, this means the provision of teachers' courses, courses on teaching of communication skills, practice management, etc., but if this method was applied in other settings, education provision would need to be made for teams to develop the necessary skills to meet the criteria.

These principles also apply to many other forms of performance review or evaluation. Vocational training is just one example of a situation where there is a fine balance to be maintained between centrally determined targets, local contracting and management, and individual practice responsibility. It is also an example of a situation in which the profession has retained the responsibility for maintaining standards and has not shied away from some difficult decisions in individual cases. In this instance there is a defined service that a practice can apply to provide—teaching a trainee; a regulatory body with responsibility for ensuring that the service is delivered and that the consumer's needs are met; and a contract which has to be renewed every 4 years. It does not take too much imagination to envisage the ways in which this scenario could be applied to other services and other contracts, and this could be a very positive or an extremely damaging development.

Joint Committee visiting

The same principles could be applied to the visiting of regions by representatives of the Joint Committee on Postgraduate Education for General Practice. At the start, the criteria used related largely to training practices, which were meant to serve as proxy measure of the regional organization and effectiveness. There are now criteria that relate directly to the performance of the regional advisors themselves. The panel of visitors currently does not include all associate advisors, and visitors do not receive much training or feedback.

CONCLUSIONS

Evaluation is all about change, and people are much more likely to change if they are involved in reviewing their own work and deciding the need to change. This is the reason for emphasizing the more democratic methods of evaluation in this chapter.

Evaluation is also central to the task of assuring the quality of education.

Ensuring that evaluation is conducted in ways that are sufficiently rigorous to be effective is the responsibility of all those concerned with, and responsible for, quality.

Those responsible for vocational training should:

- consider what questions evaluation could answer;
- understand what methods are available;
- review the means by which the release courses are evaluated;
- review the training practice approvals.

Appendix V sets out the Oxford Trainer Approval Criteria.

Part 3

12 Opportunities for the future

In this chapter we look back to previous parts of the book to draw together the main themes and look forward to how these should influence the development of vocational training in the future.

Vocational training needs to equip doctors to cope with the future demands of primary care, and enable them to help shape that future. The environment that these new doctors are entering needs to change, and training practices can provide professional leadership. For these reasons it is essential to have a clear vision for primary care, and to consider its educational implications.

We want to emphasize that many things that we have discussed in Part 2 can be done now to improve training within the existing structures. However, training could be even more effective if changes are made in the infrastructure and organization, so finally we will make our case for more radical reform.

PRIMARY CARE IN THE FUTURE

The development of a health-care system based on primary care is one of the main achievements of the National Health Service, and in the recent reforms primary care has again been recognized by the Department of Health as the foundation for future development.

It is important that although this builds on the outstanding achievements of the past, care must also continue to adapt to alterations in the environment, the new structure of the health service (NHS Management Executive 1991), and changes in society. Continuity and evolution should be emphasized to avoid both unnecessary disruption of many good working practices and the loss of the unique features which have contributed to the achievements so far. A number of themes are apparent in the evolution of primary care which will continue to be of paramount importance for practitioners in the future.

Personal accessible and continuing care

The provision of care to individuals by either a personal doctor or by identified members of a team has been a crucial feature in the aspirations of general practitioners and a highly prized asset for patients (Cartwright and Anderson 1981). This personal doctoring is both rewarding and personally demanding, and, if it is to be maintained, teachers need to ensure that doctors are appropriately equipped for it.

The traditional needs of patients for care for undifferentiated problems will remain a prime concern of both doctors and their patients. The skills of the generalist who is able to respond to these will remain a high priority. Such skills include those of diagnosis in physical, psychological, and social terms, management within primary care where appropriate, and referral when necessary.

Provision of a defined range of services

However, if primary care is to play a central role in the care of patients, and to meet the full range of their needs, it will no longer be possible for practices to opt out of other core areas, such as chronic disease management or family planning. Practices will therefore have to guarantee to provide an agreed range of services. This is different from the present situation where practitioners are, to a greater or lesser extent, free to decide for themselves both the type and level of service that they will provide. The implications are that training also cannot choose to ignore some areas and that the needs of patients will determine its content, rather than the preferences of teachers or learners.

Care of a defined population

One of the unique features of the National Health Service is the 'list system', with most of the population having an identified provider of primary care and records that follow the patient. This offers the possibility of providing a wider range of services and ensuring optimal health care for all patients, together with unique opportunities for research. The system also allows the development of provisions for prevention of illness and the promotion of health for the population as well as for individuals within it. However, it imposes on general practitioners and primary health-care teams the responsibility of ensuring equity of provision for all members of their practice population.

It also creates the opportunity to undertake assessments of need for sections of the population. These assessments can inform decisions about the purchasing of secondary care and the range of services that should be provided within primary care. General practitioners will need to be able to contribute to health-care planning and to develop the necessary negotiating and political skills required to do so. There will also be a greater need to develop the skills of population medicine and an understanding of the epidemiological principles involved (Morrell 1989).

Health promotion

The case for promoting health and preventing disease in primary care was made by the Royal College of General Practitioners in 1981, and there is every indication that both government and patients now increasingly expect GPs to be active in this field. The challenge is to make programmes effective, both in terms of their coverage of at-risk groups and in the interventions offered. This requires the skills of individual counselling as well as the ability to work with other professionals, groups, and the community.

These themes will continue to need the continuing development of the attributes of good practice that are already emerging.

Teamwork

The increasing expectations of patients, governments, and the profession can only be met by greater interdependence of members of the primary health-care team. At the same time, the increasing professionalism of other members of the team, such as practice nurses, demands recognition. Important issues requiring new attitudes and skills are already clear. These include those of communication between members of teams, identification and respect for various roles, and attention to the relationship between them.

Practice management

It is already clear that practices need effective management and that, while professional managers have an extremely important contribution to make to the development of primary health-care teams, general practitioners cannot opt out of their role as managers, whether or not the present structure of independently contracting practices is maintained. Management skills will therefore remain an extremely important aspect of the attributes of future general practitioners.

Managing change

Many of the changes envisaged in this chapter are already in train in many practices, although the pace of change varies widely. Other imminent developments are potentially of great importance. These include new techniques for investigation and treatment of disease, and new opportunities for disease prevention. However, the main challenge remains the implementation of knowledge, skills, and attitudes already present.

This is particularly important at a time when the profession has been subjected to radical changes of varying utility, which have been imposed with little regard to the principles of change management. The management of change in relation to training should both ensure that it is useful and also be a model for learners, for whom this is a key part of their training.

Information technology

A flow of reliable information will be required to support many of the changes envisaged. The current system of medical records, which forms such a significant part of caring for individuals and groups in the population, is increasingly being held on computers. In the near future practice computer systems will also have the potential to offer support for decision making and to enable the evaluation of quality of care. Practice computers will be able to network with the systems used by other workers in primary care and in hospitals. At the very least, general practitioners will need to be able to use a computer, and ideally be able to understand their potential contributions and make decisions about their application in practice.

Accountability

The general climate of accountability and the particular interest in the quality of medical care in the population will continue to put a high priority on the need for quality assurance. It is axiomatic that clinical practice should be in line with current evidence and this implies skills in obtaining information about best practice, including reading and critical thought. At the same time there is every likelihood that financial restrictions will remain or increase, with the result that value for money will need to be demonstrated. Such audit will need to embrace all the professionals working in primary care on an equal footing and to be focused on the care of patients both as individuals and in groups. The ability to initiate programmes of quality assurance, including audit, is therefore an important skill for the future.

Self-care

The expectations of professionals and patients alike and the rapid rate of change impose enormous pressures on the members of primary health-care teams. The medical profession has been prominent amongs those showing stress-related disorders, and there is evidence of deteriorating mental health amongst general practitioners following the implementation of the new contract (Sutherland and Cooper 1992). It is therefore essential that as primary care evolves the arrangements give proper emphasis to individuals taking care of themselves and to teams accepting responsibility for the well-being of their members.

Implications

These features of primary care need to be reflected with appropriate emphasis in the education of future general practitioners. It may be argued that for some doctors working in general practice, training in the clinical tasks would be sufficient, and that the more managerial tasks could be learnt later. However, unless entrants into general practice understand the principles involved in management, they would not have equal status in practice and this could lead to a very different, two-tier, career structure. This would create the need for further professional training, and might enable the appointment of 'managing partners'. At the present time the aim in vocational training is to equip trainees to play a full part in the practices they enter.

Meeting these challenges will have implications for training practices, trainers, hospital departments, vocational training schemes, trainees themselves, and regional advisers.

The prominence given to primary care in the future of the health service and the changes currently under way offer opportunities for developments, many of which can be achieved now without major structural changes.

EDUCATIONAL PRINCIPLES

It is now possible to relate the demands placed on training by the future development of primary care to the educational principles described in the earlier parts of this book.

Planned curriculum

If the general practitioner in the future is going to need an even wider repertoire of skills, and patients are to be assured that a full range of services are provided, then the curriculum for training is large. It needs to be defined explicitly in the light of both the present needs and future requirements of general practice. This is the task of individual trainers, training schemes, and those responsible for the certification of the completion of training. The success of vocational training in the past has rested largely on the individual enthusiasm and commitment of innovative teachers and their learners. This energy needs harnessing to achieve the breadth of learning required to meet the needs in future, while not losing the dynamism of a developing discipline.

Another implication is that the curriculum will need to focus more on generic skills rather than specific content, particularly those skills that will help the doctor to cope with changing practice, for example interpersonal and management skills.

Effective use of time

There is also an imperative to use the time available for training as effectively as possible. It is apparent that there is a wide disparity between theoretical considerations and the educational experience of many trainees. One reason for this is the relative lack of priority given to educational aspects of training posts. Educational considerations are seldom made explicit, and the aims, methods, and assessment arrangements are rarely defined. Another aspect of this is the balance of experience and learning. Many of the assumptions that underlie the current approach to educational posts rely on the perceived value of repeated experiences without adequate opportunity to reflect on, and learn from, that experience. The optimal balance of experience and learning should be based on the learning needs of individuals, not just the service needs of patients.

Many of the difficulties currently experienced by trainees are due to the failure to exploit the opportunities offered by the 3 years of vocational training. In some cases this is because the doctor's career path has not been decided, and special arrangements need to be made for such individuals. However, for the majority of intending GPs, there is a much greater potential in a 3 year period than is presently realized. The definition of learning objectives and the recording of their achievement through such mechanisms as log books should ensure a more systematic approach both to specific objectives and to use of the time available.

Learner-centred teaching

Much of this book has emphasized the need to recognize the implications of working with adult learners. This has been seen mainly through the eyes of trainers and their practices, but much the same considerations apply to learning in hospital posts. Our experience and the lessons from educational theory suggest that our methods should be looked at critically in order to make sure that they are tailored, as far as possible, both to a developing professional at particular stages in his or her career and to his or her individual needs.

It is important that the learner and the teacher share the responsibility for the learning. Sharing the responsibility does not mean that either side can abrogate their part. Learner-centred approaches still require the trainer to bring and negotiate an agenda, which may be a more demanding task than simply following the trainee.

Multidisciplinary education

General practitioners already use methods that were developed in other disciplines, including psychology, nursing, management, and education. In some cases these have been taught by practitioners from those fields, but too often this is not so. There may have been an ethos which encouraged the view that doctors should only be taught by other doctors. Not only may this limit the access of trainees to different ideas and expertise; it prevents young doctors from appreciating the potential contribution that others can make to primary care.

If isolation from other professionals can be partly overcome by learning from them, it can also be reduced by learning together. Experience with working with mixed groups from various disciplines suggests that this can increase understanding and may be a much surer basis for the teamworking that will be needed in the future.

IMPLICATIONS FOR TRAINING PRACTICES AND TRAINERS

There will be a number of implications for trainers and training practices.

Training practices vary in their level of 'busyness'. Part of this variation is due to different levels and styles of management, but part of it is due to workload. It is clear that unless priority is given to educational activities, these become swamped, and in the future it will be increasingly unacceptable for education to be squeezed out of a position of importance. There should therefore be enough time, not only for tutorials between trainers and trainees, but also for educational meetings within the practice and for the practice to be involved in discussions about trainees' progress. Trainees need protected time for reading, case studies, and projects, but trainers also need time for preparation, planning and reflection. The fundamental requirement is a commitment from all the partners to being an effective teaching practice. Any practice should be able to give as much time to educational activities as the trainee spends seeing the GPs patients.

Teaching practices have an important part to play both in the development of individual trainees and in the development of the profession as a whole. The importance of modelling has been stressed, and therefore teachers must offer high standards both in the conduct of their profession and also in education. In the early days of vocational training, emphasis was placed on high professional standing, but less on the educational aspects. An equal balance now needs to be achieved. This implies increasing attention both to the past and future educational achievements of trainers, who should be encouraged to study for higher qualifications.

Audit or quality assurance will be increasingly important in the future. Mechanisms must be in place in training practices to demonstrate their own effectiveness and to act as examples to doctors in training.

The importance of teamworking has already been stressed. However, if it is to be effective, it will need to be demonstrated with in the practice and in the educational process. The use of practice staff to teach the trainee on an equal footing with the doctors is an important demonstration of principle and a way of allowing the education to benefit from wider inputs. Shared teaching and learning with, for example, nursing, health visiting, and social work students can take place within the practice. Attempts have been made in the past to identify practices as multidisciplinary learning environments, but these have not always been successful. The reasons for the lack of success, however, have usually been administrative rather than educational or professional, and such initiatives should continue to be pursued if possible.

Everything that has been said rests on the assumption that trainers will keep themselves up to date and will also update their teaching skills. A commitment to such learning is therefore extremely important for the trainer, and the support of this must be one of the duties of training practices. Other members of the team involved in teaching may also wish to have the opportunity to develop their teaching skills, and multidisciplinary teaching courses might be a very valuable way forward.

IMPLICATIONS FOR TRAINING SCHEMES

A vocational training scheme offers a variety of possible learning experiences, but time is limited. It is therefore important that these experiences are co-ordinated. In particular, the roles of the practices and various courses need to be examined so that overlaps are minimized or are used in a constructive way. The organization of training on 3 year schemes is, at least theoretically, based on the concept of a comprehensive programme. A strong case has been made in Chapter 10 for the involvement of course organizers in the planning of these programmes, and this is already occurring some places.

If the curriculum is more clearly defined, then it would be possible for trainees to have personal logs to record their experience, and their performance in each post could be assessed against the learning objectives for that post.

The main strength of training schemes lies in the trainers and the training practices. The maintenance of their enthusiasm and the contribution that they make is crucial. This will depend on their active involvement in developments in the scheme, giving trainers recognition and support, and providing courses for trainers that enable them to develop their teaching skills as well as their knowledge of the curriculum.

If the case for the wider curriculum described earlier is accepted, it may be reasonable to expect each training practice to exemplify all its aspects; for example, high-quality patient care, effective management, and teamwork. However, it is unrealistic to expect each trainer and course organizer to understand the background and theory required to teach all aspects themselves. It may be that special skills will need to develop within trainers' groups, with different trainers taking responsibility for different areas.

In the first instance, it may be more feasible for the scheme rather than individual practices to forge links with training schemes for other disciplines, such as nurses, health visitors, and social workers, and to arrange joint teaching sessions. In the longer term it may be possible to develop multidisciplinary training practices with team teaching and learning.

IMPLICATIONS FOR TRAINEES

The main thrust of this book has been to base the development of education for general practice on the principles of adult education. Principally, our concerns have been to ensure an appropriate structure and skill base to support this. However, active participation by the learner will be an essential ingredient of the recommended approach to education. Changes occurring in undergraduate and postgraduate education may facilitate this change.

Some undergraduate education is becoming more problem based, and this will create a climate that will empower young doctors to play a greater part in their own learning. The importance of communication skills and personal development is also being recognized, and the GMC has recommended greater emphasis on health promotion and on learning in the community.

Postgraduate training is dependent on the earlier education of future GPs and the quality of those recruited. There is a range of attitudes to general practice in the undergraduate programmes in the United Kingdom. Much of traditional medical education is based on a specialist systematic approach, while some of the recently established schools take a more holistic approach. This stereotype is not wholly true, since long-established institutions have recently changed considerably and there are younger organizations that follow a traditional model. There are two important issues for vocational training. In the first instance, trainers should be aware of the different approaches to the undergraduate curriculum, especially in relation to skills such as those needed for communications. Secondly, the whole emphasis of training programmes will need to be sensitive to the attributes that had been acquired by doctors prior to entry.

There is increasing acceptance that the educational purpose of pre-registration and SHO posts should be clearly stated, and that more attention should be given to doctors' personal and emotional needs during this time. Doctors entering vocational training will then be better prepared to recognize their own learning needs and to discuss ways in which these can be met.

IMPLICATIONS FOR POSTGRADUATE ORGANIZATIONS

Finally, the implementation of these changes will require the active support of advisers and the postgraduate education committee structure. They have a responsibility to provide a clear strategy for the development of training. They also appoint trainers and course organizers, allocate budgets, and can provide courses for trainers and sometimes for trainees as well.

There is a great need for appropriate leadership that recognizes the expertise that exists at all levels, especially in the training practices and local schemes. The challenge is, therefore, to find structures and processes that do not inhibit development, but which help to channel the enthusiasm of trainers, course organizers, and advisers. This implies a dynamic relationship between the centre and periphery, both locally and nationally.

A balance between bottom-up and top-down approaches has to be struck. On the one hand, those working at the centre have legitimate claims to influencing policy, given their potential for a broader view of what is happening locally and elsewhere. On the other hand, they must not become isolated from those involved in the practical work of education, or lose sight of the constraints on trainers and course organizers, the needs of particular situations or individuals, and the value of innovations. Where possible, we suggest that the boundaries, requirements, and objectives should be set by the central group, but that the methods of delivery of any particular objective should be the prerogative of courses and training practices. The principle of what is known as 'subsidiarity' in Euro-speak should apply in training as in macro-political structures. In addition, when creating this strategic framework, the views of individual trainers and course organizers should be taken fully into account. This may be achieved through a variety of mechanisms, including established trainers' groups or workshops, and through *ad hoc* representative groups set up for specific purposes. Those who are selected to lead the development of training need to have vision, and to be able to help others share in that vision by challenge, support, and by constructing effective dialogue.

The criteria for the appointment of trainers should reflect the educational considerations already described, and trainers need to be fully committed to these criteria and involved in the selection process. Approximately one in four practices in the United Kingdom are training practices. If the methods of assessment and approval are designed to promote development both of the practice and of the teaching, there is a major opportunity to have a positive influence on the directions of change.

Trainers' courses should also contribute to the achievement of the overall strategy and should address both the methods and the content of training. For example, if the aim is to develop the teaching of management skills, then trainers may want courses on both the practice of management, and on its theory, together with ways that it can be taught effectively.

In most parts of the country, course organizers will be the pivot around which educational change will take place. They therefore have to be recruited carefully, offered appropriate training, and their progress reviewed on a regular basis. If the strategy is to promote critical thinking and audit, course organizers and GP tutors should be expected to take some form of higher degree, such as an M.Sc. or Dip.Ed., and to have produced some published work.

THE ORGANIZATION OF VOCATIONAL TRAINING IN THE FUTURE

The development of vocational training within a space of 30 years has been one of the outstanding achievements in medical education and an important factor in the current key position of primary care in the NHS. However, its organization evolved from existing structures and inevitably a number of compromises had to be made.

We have argued that much can be done to improve training within the present structure. However, to realize fully the potential of vocational training it will require changes to its organization, and in education for primary care more generally.

Academic departments of primary care

The academic side of primary care is fragmented, with separate undergraduate departments of general practice, vocational training schemes, and continued medical education. It is also isolated from those working in a variety of other institutions, such as schools of nursing and colleges of higher education. We have suggested that trainees should be taught by, and learn with, other professionals. This will only be achieved by much greater co-operation, either on a functional basis or through new structures such as institutes of primary care. Changes of this nature will require different attitudes amongst teachers, but also support from institutions and financial resources to provide the appropriate physical environment. These new departments would be able to develop expertise both in medical education and in research in primary care.

Different standards have also come to apply in the selection and recruitment of doctors who teach in different settings. At a higher level, the division between advisers and professors also embodies the split. This could be remedied by unified departments with leadership shared, possibly on a rotating basis, between undergraduate and postgraduate wings, if these persist. In order for this to occur, there will need to be a common acceptance of the need for higher qualifications for all involved in academic general practice.

Educational evaluation

Some of the success of vocational training has been due to collaborations between medical teachers and educationalists, which have led to the introduction of teaching methods developed in other fields but new to medicine, including some of the ideas in this book. However, many of the methods currently used have not been evaluated, and meeting the new challenges will require methods that will need evaluating in their own turn. There is also a need to evaluate the process of training in terms of its validity as a preparation for general practice; an effective academic department would include members with a particular interest in evaluation.

The status of 'trainees'

The success of vocational training to date has rested largely on the enthusiasm and commitment of innovative teachers and their learners, particularly in the early days of voluntary training. These created a momentum which sustained both individuals and the emerging system. It is essential that this is maintained, and that trainers have the time and the support that they require.

The pattern of training, with trainees employed by one trainer for a year, works well if the relationship, the practice, and the teaching are all satisfactory. On the other hand, it limits the range of experience for the trainee, creates the expectation that they will spend much of their time working as an assistant in the practice, and the scope of the training depends on the limitations of the individual trainer and practice. If the needs are for a more consistent curriculum and the effective use of time, it would be more effective for trainees to be employed by the postgraduate or academic department, the length and nature of their practice attachments being determined by their educational needs.

The transfer of 50 per cent of the salary of SHOs to the budget of post-graduate deans is a recognition of the importance of purchasing appropriate education in these posts. The employment of trainees by the academic or postgraduate department would represent an extension of the same principle into the general practice component of training. We would also welcome the transfer of the remaining 50 per cent of the budget for SHOs to the educational budget.

It would also be appropriate to change the title 'trainee' to one that recognizes the educational purpose of the post, but avoids the connotations of subservience associated with it. We suggest adopting the title 'registrar' because the status and the role would be recognized in other branches of the profession.

The length of training

The Royal Commission on Postgraduate Medical Education, reporting in 1968, proposed that training for general practice should last for 5 years. Although alterations in undergraduate education and better use of the pre-registration year may mean that entrants to training may be better prepared, there will continue to be enormous pressure on time during training. Therefore the split between general professional and general practice training, the balance between hospital and practice experience, and the overall length of the training period all need review.

The Cairns report has proposed a period of general professional training between pre-registration posts and specialist training (REF). If this occurred, it would be an opportunity to gain clinical experience and develop generic skills that will be valuable to all new general practitioners. Discussions about training and the development of primary care often reveal a lack of understanding amongst hospital doctors, and this would be reduced if all doctors had a period in general practice as part of general professional training for all specialities.

It may well be that specialist training for general practice will still need to include further hospital experience in relevant departments. However, most commentators have highlighted the incongruity of a training programme for general practice that takes place in hospitals for 2 out of the 3 years. Whatever the duration of vocational training in the future, it is important that more than 12 months can be spent in practice. This is already possible under the regulations for training, but is prevented by the arrangements for funding. An extension of training in general practice would allow much greater preparation of trainees, especially in the areas of management. Experience of such arrangements has been obtained in experimental schemes in Northampton and Dartford in the 1970s, which were regarded as a success. Reference has been made to the need for more flexibility in the future, and this should certainly apply to this balance. Flexibility must allow for the period of training to be determined by the needs of the doctor in training, as determined by both formative and summative assessment, and it may be most appropriate to specify only a minimum period.

Further education in practice

Young general practitioners have special needs in their early years in practice. These are partly due to the need for support as they adjust to new environments, and partly due to gaps in their training, particularly in the area of practice management. Young practitioners groups are a valuable source of support, but they cannot provide the additional educational resources needed. Several educational solutions have already been explored to address the needs of this group of doctors, including our own activities at Oxford (Baillon *et al.* 1993). Courses aimed at new principals have generally attracted only a small number of enthusiastic members, who would probably be better served by a course leading to a higher degree. The majority of new general practitioners do not undertake courses because of the disincentives, including the lack of protected time for education and an understandable desire to get on with the job. A new initiative to support education into the early years in practice would involve changes in its status, including tying it to a system of recertification, and providing more financial support for time spent on educational activities.

More radically, we may see changes in the career structure of general practice, with a different type of post between trainee and established partner—perhaps akin to the senior registrar grade in hospital. This would encourage more mobility and career progression, but might be open to exploitation. An alternative may be to have two grades of principal, with the facility for further training and assessment leading to progress from one grade to the next.

CONCLUSION

In this final chapter we have attempted to argue that our task is to prepare doctors for their future in primary care, that looking to that future we can identify some clear trends now but we can be certain that the pace of change will continue. We can apply the educational principles described earlier in the book to design a vocational training that meets this challenge. Many of the required developments in our training practices, our courses, and in our teaching can be achieved now if we have the determination to make them.

However, structural change is also essential. Without it, it will not be possible to realize the full potential of education for the general practitioners who will play a key role in the primary care system on which depends the future of the National Health Service.

Appendix I Priority objectives for Vocational Training

This appendix was originally published as Chapter 3 of Occasional Paper 30 of the Royal College of General Practitioners (1988). It is reproduced by permission of the RCGP.

We have described five areas in which the general practitioner needs to be competent: patient care, communication, organization, professional values, and personal and professional growth. We now need to consider and select specific educational objectives for each area. In making this selection we have tried to apply a number of principles.

PRINCIPLES OF SELECTION

The first is to select those objectives which are crucial to the doctor's work, for example, the ability to deal effectively with life-threatening illness and the ability to communicate with patients. Secondaly, we consider those attitudes and skills that are commonly required in a large proportion of the doctor's work. Thirdly, we have given priority to attributes that are not only required now but will continue to be required throughout a doctor's professional life-time and particularly the ability to review his own work and to adapt to and produce change. Finally, we have given priority to understanding principles or developing skills that can be transferred from the condition or setting in which they are learned to other settings and conditions in the future. This is educationally effective and more economical.

Though the list of priority objectives may look long, we have tried to make them specific, which . . . should make them easier for teachers to apply. We emphasize once again, however, that they are not intended as a list of tutorials to be worked through. Vocational training extends over three years and takes place in hospital and general practice, supplemented by day release courses and other teaching. Therefore, these objectives may be achieved in any of these places and it is up to course organizers and trainers to decide when they introduce topics and how much time each individual trainee need on each section. The implications of this are discussed in the final chapter.

PATIENT CARE

One of the difficulties facing a general practitioner is the wide range of problems with which he has to deal and this means it is virtually impossible to draw up a list of conditions that all trainees should be competent to manage by the end of training. All trainees will see a wide, but not necessarily adequate, range of problems during their training programme and we believe the essential objectives are largely to do with general principles, which can be learned from some problems which have been seen and subsequently applied to others which have not. Those doctors wanting a detailed list of conditions, together with their frequency, will find it in the Oxford Region General Practice Training Curriculum Guide available in the Medical School offices.

1. *Problem definition*
The doctor should be able to demonstrate that he:

(a) can recognize common physical, psychological and social problems presenting in general practice and give equal consideration to them;

(b) can include in his assessment of the problem:

- the patient's beliefs, ideas and concerns about the problem
- its effects on daily living, family and friends
- its effects on the psychological state of the patient
- the patient's expectations of the doctor.

(c) understands the principles of problem definition, including:

- the consideration of appropriate possibilities
- the use of probabilities
- the use of selective history taking, physical examination and investigations.

(d) can cope with his own anxieties, particularly in relation to:

- the unstructured presentation
- the inability to reach a firm conclusion
- the lack of continual professional monitoring.

2. *Management*
The doctor should be able to demonstrate in his management of the patient's problem that he:

(a) can choose with the patient the appropriate management for each problem;

(b) understands the importance of making and reassesing a management plan which includes:

- the effective involvement of other members of the team
- the effective use of records.

(c) in his prescribing of drugs, has a knowledge of their:

- pharmacological action
- side effects
- interactions

- dosage
- cost
- regulations, including that of scheduled drugs
- appropriate use

and that he is aware of the sources of information concerning other drugs.

(d) has the knowledge and skills necessary for the management of life events and crises. These include, for example, death, alcoholism, domestic upheavals and psychiatric illness.
(e) can provide appropriate care and support for his patients and their families.
(f) has the knowledge of available agencies and resources, and skills to make appropriate referrals.
(g) understands the importance of appropriate involvement and education of the patient.
(h) is aware of the costs of his activities, especially in the field of prescribing, and practises in the knowledge that the resources of health care are finite.

3. *Emergency care*
The doctor should be able to diagnose and initially manage in general practice all acute emergency situations and provide immediate follow-up care where appropriate. Important examples of these are acute asthma, pulmonary embolus, myocardial infarction, acute left ventricular failure, acute abdomen, acute haemorrhage, management of the unconscious patient, including diabetic coma and hypoglycaemic coma, status epilepticus, road traffic accident, obstructed airway, self-poisoning, acute depression and compulsory mental health admission.

4. *Prevention*
The doctor should be able to demonstrate that he:

(a) understands the principles involved in identifying preventable diseases in general practice, for example:

- case finding during routine consultations
- health education during routine consultations
- screening sub-groups of the population
- monitoring preventive activities, e.g. immunization and cervical screening rates; level of family planning; attendance at child health development clinics; health education for groups of patients and the community at large.

(b) has a knowledge of systems used to identify individuals and sections of the practice population.
(c) is able to provide effective preventive services to individual patients and to his registered practice population.

COMMUNICATION

1. *Patients*
Communication with patients takes place largely in the consulting room but also at home, on the telephone, and in other situations. Effective communication can be defined as the ability to establish or maintain a relationship with the patient and to use appropriate strategies and skills to achieve the aims of patient care.

The tasks that can be achieved in a consultation have . . . been described by Pendleton *et al.* (1984) and have been incorporated in our objectives for patient care. The doctor should be able to demonstrate that he can achieve these tasks in his consultations.

2. *Partners, practice team and other professionals*
The doctor should be able to demonstrate:

(a)   understanding and respect for the professional training and differing roles of members of the practice team and other disciplines who may be involved in the care of his/her patients. This is particularly important in relation to:

- district nursing sisters
- treatment room sisters
- health visitors
- community midwives
- social workers
- practice managers, secretaries and receptionists.

(b)   his understanding of the importance of meetings and discussion with his partners, family, practice team, and local colleagues in hospitals and general practice.
(c)   the skill to discover the strengths and weaknesses of the members of these groups and their need for support.
(d)   the use of his knowledge of the practice and his patients to their mutual benefit in various contacts, such as at practice meetings, team meetings, on the telephone, at interdisciplinary meetings, and within the family.

ORGANIZATION

We emphasize the need to be able to monitor and manage as being more important initially than being conversant with every paragraph in the Statement of Fees and Allowances (Red Book). If the broad principles are grasped, it is likely much else will follow . . .

1. *The practice*
The doctor should be able to demonstrate:

(a) an understanding of the importance of the need manage a practice effectively.

(b) an ability to monitor aspects of practice activity, including:

- accessibility and appointment systems
- information given to patients
- records and registers
- employment and attachment of staff
- use of time.

(c) the ability to take appropriate action when problems are identified in these fields.

(d) his knowledge of the most important sections of the NHS contract and regulations, including:

- his principle obligations
- sources of income
- superannuation.

(e) his knowledge of the most important organizational aspects of practice and partnership, including:

- partnership agreements
- principles of book-keeping and accounts
- financing of premises
- income tax.

(f) his understanding of the application of new technology to general practice.

(g) his understanding of the principles of the successful introduction of change and innovation including:

- the nature of innovation
- the characteristics of the adopter
- the characteristics of the organization
- the implications for his future practice.

2. *Personal*
(a) The doctor should be able to demonstrate the ability to manage his time:

- in consultations
- in the balance between patient care, the practice, his family and other activities.

(b) The doctor should demonstrate an awareness of his own limitations, respect the skills of others, and the ability to delegate appropriately.

3. *Community*
(a) The doctor should be able to determine and to respond to the health needs of the community.
(b) He must know how and where to intervene in the community on behalf of individuals or groups of patients and have the ability to deal with and relate to a wide range of people responsible for community affairs.

PROFESSIONAL VALUES

In this section we have attempted to describe some personal attitudes and values which we regard as fundamental attributes of the good general practitioner.

The doctor should be able to demonstrate:

(a) awareness of his own values, beliefs and attitudes, the factors that influence them, and the way that they affect his work and relationships with patients and colleagues.
(b) his recognition of the social, cultural, and organizational factors that define and affect his work as a doctor (e.g. social class, race, methods of payment).
(c) the possession and application of ethical principles in his work. These include:

- respect for the value of human life
- respect for the dignity of patients and the promotion of their autonomy
- maintenance of confidentiality
- willingness broadly to place the needs of the patients above his own convenience
- justice and fairness in allocating resources
- personal and professional integrity.

(d) tolerance, respect and flexibility in his response to the ideas of others, including those of his patients, peers and teachers.
(e) his willingness to submit his work to review by his peers and the ability to give and receive criticism.
(f) that he is able to maintain his own physical and mental health. He should be aware of the stresses of his work and of his own responses and defence mechanisms. He should be able to seek and obtain appropriate support.
(g) his awareness of the factors that influence the relationships between his personal and professional life (e.g. financial and family commitments).
(h) a willingness to accept appropriate responsibility for his patients, partners and colleagues within the practice. He should be prepared to provide appropriate support for others in the practice.

	Content of curriculum	Method of learning	Assessment method
The practitioner	Protocols • formulation • introduction • evaluation Auditing practice care • individual patients • BP and smoking clinics • the practice population Teamwork New technology Health education in the community Setting up a BP clinic Handling change Presentational skills	Literature Team discussion and meetings Project work An audit Presentation of results Tutorials • doctors • nurses • managers • others Visits to other practices	See methods of learning MCQ MEQ Mid-term assessment (external) Self-assessment rating scales

Appendix IV Teamwork: an example of staging

	Entry criteria	Method of learning	Assessment method
The new trainee	The trainee selection process • curriculum vitae • references • structured questionaire • interview personal attributes ability to work in a team compatibility with partners flexibility motivation (to learn)	A structured introductory programme Negotiating the next stage	Encounter sheets • information gathering • decision making • recording results Analysis
The practising trainee	'The trainee understands the roles of the team' Credentials of team members established Knowledge of how the team works Acceptance of and by the team	Participation • joint care of patients • participation in team meetings • case discussion Modelling • example • osmosis • sharing of craft knowledge Project Involvement in change management	Feedback from all team members • written • verbal MEQ Observation by trainer with recorded information Analysis and negotiation of future programme

	Entry criteria	Method of learning	Assessment method
The practitioner	'The trainee is accepted as a new team member' The theoretical background of teamwork is understood	Experience in • co-operating • leading • delegating • motivating self and others	External • MRCGP • MEQ Internal • MEQ • case analysis Self • Manchester rating scales • critical thinking • audit
	'The trainee becomes an effective member of the team'		

Appendix V Criteria for the approval of trainers and training practices (Oxford) (Schofield and Hasler 1984)

INTRODUCTION

These criteria were drawn up by a working party of trainers and course organisers, and have been discussed by all the trainers' groups and endorsed by the General Practice Subcommittee in the Oxford Region. These criteria are based on requirements for teaching and are not intended to define the 'ideal general practice'. No trainer or teaching practice will fulfil all the criteria completely at any one time. The criteria do, however, indicate the areas and directions that trainers and teaching practices should continue to develop to improve the opportunities they offer their trainees. These criteria are used as the basis for the approval and reapproval of trainers and training practices, and these assessments will take into account both the level of performance in each area at the time, and also the progress that is being made towards achieving them more completely.

The responsibility for the approval of trainers rests with the General Practice Subcommittee (Para 38.1 SFA), and the members are guided by national guidelines laid down by the Joint Committee on Postgraduate Training for General Practice.

Those criteria that are mandatory are set in bold type.

A. STATEMENT OF PRINCIPLE

Teaching practices and trainers are selected for the educational opportunities that they offer to their trainees. Trainees may learn from (a) experience and example working in the training practices; (b) teaching from the trainer; (c) the other educational resources and opportunities available in the practice. All these areas must therefore be examined in the approval process.

Each teaching practice is part of the regional and district training schemes. It should subscribe to the regional aims for training and contribute appropriately to its district scheme. The responsibility for the education of each individual trainee in the practice, however, remains with that trainee and trainer.

B. THE TRAINER

1. Professional values

The trainer should be a doctor committed to providing a high standard of care for his patients. He should believe in the importance of continuity of care, give a personal service and try to make it as comprehensive as possible. He should balance his own convenience against that of his patients and keep the interests of the wider community in mind. He should be of good repute and known for his integrity and have good relationships with his colleagues and staff. He should encourage patients' self-help and keep in balance his need to be needed. His clinical decisions should reflect the true long-term interests of his patients. He should see himself as providing a service to his practice population, sharing with others the responsibility for promoting, preserving and restoring the health of the individual patients. Trainers should not display racial or sexual prejudice either in their practices or their training.

2. Previous experience

A trainer must have at least five years' experience as a principal general practitioner.

3. Clinical competence

The trainer should display a high standard of clinical competence in his consultations, the long-term care of patients, preventative medicine, prescribing, record keeping, auditing his own work, and appropriate use of other members of the practice health care team and of colleagues in agencies outside.

4. Continuing education

The trainer subjects his work to critical self-scrutiny and peer review and accepts a commitment to keep up to date, to improve his skills and widen his range of services in response to newly disclosed needs. **He must fulfil the annual requirements for the postgraduate educational allowance.**

5. Preparation for teaching

Before initial appointment, a trainer must have attended an approved course for new trainers and have participated regularly in the meetings of the local trainers group for at least six months. Attendance at a course for consultation skills and visiting other training practices is also recommended.

He must be familiar with educational aims for vocational training and methods of teaching and assessment.

New trainers must have passed the MRCGP examination. This demonstrates a willingness to be assessed and preparation for the examination is also valuable preparation for teaching. The trainer should also be to help the trainee prepare to sit the MRCGP examination at the end of vocational training.

6. Continuing commitment to teaching

The trainer will regard teaching and meeting the educational needs of his trainee as a major commitment. This will be reflected in time, enthusiasm, and the desire to develop as a professional teacher. He should be aware of new ideas and developments in general practice and with the main literature of general practice. **By the end of his first two years approval he must have attended a course for the general development of his teaching skills which includes communication and consultation skills. Thereafter he must attend appropriate courses for trainers (within or outside the region) every four years**.

7. Contribution to the local scheme and to the region

A trainer must belong and contribute to the local trainers' group. He should be willing to work with, to support and be supported by colleagues in the development of teaching. He should be prepared to assist and support the Course Organiser with the organisation of the scheme including help with the day-release course where appropriate. After appointment he will be invited to become a member of a visiting panel for assessment of trainers in other parts of the region and *this invitation must be accepted after two years if he continues to be appointed as a trainer*.

C. Learning and teaching

1. Relationships

The trainer should be able to develop and maintain an open, honest relationship with his trainee and generate enthusiasm and motivation in the trainee. He should have the ability to understand his trainee's problems and to communicate with the trainee. He should demonstrate an ability for logical and critical thought and willingness and ability to encourage the trainee to direct his own learning.

2. Assessment and curriculum planning

The trainer must be familiar with the Oxford Region Priority Objectives of General Practice Vocational Training (RCGP Occ Paper 30). The trainer and

trainee must jointly assess the trainee's needs at the start of the programme and these needs must be regularly reassessed during the course of the attachment. These assessments must be guided by the trainer's aims of what needs to be achieved by the end of the attachment and must cover appropriate aspects of knowledge, skills and attitudes.

The trainer and trainee must negotiate appropriate educational goals and curriculum planning in the light of these regular assessments and the trainer will need to keep in mind both short and long term aims. These must reflect the increasing confidence and competence of the trainee as well as his or her personal growth.

3. Teaching records

Records and logs must be kept by each trainer and each trainee so that it is possible to ensure that important aspects of training have been covered, that comprehensive assessments have been made and that curriculum plans are logically laid out.

A training record must be kept for each trainee for these purposes.

4. Methods

The teaching must be planned and prepared on a logical basis in relation to the educational goals. The trainer, should encourage the trainee to direct his or her own learning and to develop self awareness and critical thought. He should be able to use a variety of appropriate and effective teaching methods and be able to direct the trainee to additional resources when required.

Other members of the partnership and the primary health care team will have important contributions to make. He should encourage trainees to undertake project work, so that they can learn what is involved in reviewing and auditing care within a practice.

D. THE TEACHING PRACTICE

1. Partnership's responsibilities

The trainee needs to be accepted and treated as a colleague in the practice and involved in the work of the practice by all its members. All partners should be willing to accept the educational purpose of the trainee attachment and their own responsibilities as members of the teaching practice. These responsibilities include welcoming the trainee as a colleague and being willing to share the care of their patients. They should recognise the contribution that the trainee and the trainer make to the practice and be willing to support them and allow adequate time for their educational activities. They should also recognise the financial contribution that training makes to the practice and be willing to participate in and support the development of the practice for teaching.

2. Time for teaching and other educational activity

The trainer and partners must make adequate time available for the provision of teaching and supervision within the practice and for other outside activities for the trainer. The trainer will require the equivalent of two half-day sessions per week. The trainer and partners will need to be accessible to the trainee to discuss problems when required. **The trainer must provide uninterrupted teaching time of at least two hours a week for teaching in normal working hours.** This will normally be in one session and may be delegated usefully at times to partners and other members of the practice team. The trainee will also require the opportunity for regular joint consultations and must be free to attend courses organised outside the practice. The trainer will need time to attend the trainers' group, teachers' courses, take part in visits to other practices and scheme activities, and also time for his own educational activities.

3. List size and workload

The list size and workload of the teaching practice should be large enough to offer the trainee adequate clinical experience but not too large to prevent time being available for teaching and for attending courses both by the trainer and the trainee, or to prohibit a high standard of patient care.

4. Arrangements for seeing patients

The teaching practice should have arrangements for seeing patients, usually an appointment system, that allow adequate access of patients to the doctors, both for urgent and non-urgent problems. These arrangements should also encourage continuity of care and allow adequate time for each patient. The arrangements for a trainee to see patients should be planned to meet his educational needs. These include seeing a representative cross-section of patients, including those with long-term problems, and opportunities to establish continuing of care for patients. Trainees need to have the opportunity both to have the time to study patients and their problems in depth and also to experience working at a similar rate to the partners in practice. **Trainees must not be seeing patients at times when they do not have the opportunity to obtain advice from a partner in the practice.**

5. Night and weekend work

Arrangements for out-of-hours cover by a teaching practice should allow the on-call doctor access to information about the patients and enable him to ensure continuity of care. The trainee will require adequate experience of emergency and out-of-hours work in the practice. **When the trainee is on duty a partner in the practice must always be available to help and advise**. The trainee should not normally be expected to be on duty more often that the other partners in the practice. **The training practice is responsible for making arrangements for telephone cover while the trainee is on call**. Some practices are involved in large extended rotas or deputising services. In these circumstances the trainee should only be on call for the patients of the training practice at appropriate intervals. The trainer is also expected to be undertaking a comparable amount of out-of-hours work.

6. Medical records

The standard of medical records in a teaching practice should be sufficient to support a high standard of clinical care. These records are increasingly being held electronically as well as manually. Doctors and other members of the health team should be able to obtain necessary information rapidly and accurately.

i. **Record cards, letters, and results of investigation must be filed in chronological order after appropriate pruning**.
ii. **A legible entry must be made at each doctor–patient consultation, the management and, in particular, medication, should be clear**.
iii. **The records of all patients on regular medication must contain easily discernible drug therapy lists**. These lists can be held on computer provided that the doctor seeing the patient is aware that such a list exists and is able to access it.
iv. Each patient record should contain a medical summary or problem list. **There must be a clear and effective system for the creation and updating of these summaries and a written agreement by the practice about the content**.

Because medical records contain confidential information the GMC has advised that practices inform patients that their records may be inspected by other doctors for the purposes of education and training, and that they have a right to object if they wish to do so. This information may be provided in the form of a notice in the waiting room and in statements in practice brochures.

7. Prevention and chronic disease care

The practice must be committed to organized preventive medicine and effective chronic disease care. It therefore has to maintain age, sex, disease and other registers, which are increasingly being held electronically. The partners should be able to state what their policies are in relation to health education, case finding, screening and protocols for chronic disease care.

Prevention data in individual patient records should be easily accessible. The practice must be able to produce prevention data in relation to its population. There should be appropriate child health and developmental surveillance arrangements and effective child immunisation levels.

Data relating to chronic disease surveillance should be easily identifiable in the medical records, and guidelines for nurses, where they are providing follow-up care, should be available.

8. Performance review and medical audit

General practitioners are now required to audit their work and it is important that trainees are fully prepared to undertake this. **The practice must be committed to reviewing and auditing the care it provides for its patients**. The partners and other members of the health team should be able to demonstrate how they identify strength and weaknesses in the care of patients and how they take appropriate action to improve that care.

9. Practice premises and equipment

The premises and equipment should be adequate to allow a high standard of patient care, practice organisation and teamwork. The trainee should be able to consult in a well-equipped room and it is desirable that he or she should have a consulting room of his own. The practice should ensure that the trainee is provided with adequate equipment to carry out consultations and home visits.

10. Libraries and journals

The practice must have an organised library which is accessible to all members of the team and the trainee. The library should contain adequate up-to-date reference books, books relevant to general practice and recent copies of the major journals relevant to general practice.

11. The partnership and health care team

The practice should display a high standard of organisation and administration. **It must be committed to teamwork** and have adequate staff.

There should be close working relationships between all members of the team, both attached and employed. There needs to be regular meetings for the purposes of planning and education and it is important that all members of the team are able to raise subjects for discussion.

There will normally be a nurse working in a treatment room. The trainee should have the opportunity of participating in the work of the team and of attending special clinics, such as antenatal, child health and family planning. The trainee should also be encouraged to attend partnership and team meetings and have access to all aspects of practice management including business finance and employment.

12. Contract: letter of employment

The trainee is an employee of the training practice and must be provided with a letter of employment or written contract. This contract must not contain conditions that restrict the trainee's rights under the Statement of Fees and Allowances, or that interfere with his or her training.

13. Appointment of trainees

Trainers appointing trainees without the combined hospital and general practice scheme rotations must consult with the course organiser over the appointment and starting date. The starting dates should normally be coordinated with the starting dates in the scheme as a whole. (Oxford Regional Committee for Postgraduate Medical Education and Training.)

Appendix VI Education in training posts for junior hospital doctors (Oxford)

1. CONTENT AND PURPOSE

(a) Each training post should have a detailed job description which should include the educational content, which may have to be modified according to the experience of the holder.

(b) Junior doctors need to acquire the relevant skills in the specialty in which they are working and, at SHO level, basic skills common to all doctors. The latter (as identified by the GMC (General Medical Council 1987) include communication skills, the prevention of illness, teamwork, management, problem solving and other knowledge and skills which cross specialty boundaries. Management includes setting clinical objectives, establishing priorities, making a plan of care, deploying resources, and evaluating effectiveness of patient care.

2. SUPERVISION AND APPRAISAL

Each junior should have an identified educational supervisor (who will normally be a consultant). At the beginning of the appointment the junior should discuss and agree with his supervisor the educational objectives for his attachment (as identified in the report on Postgraduate Medical Education (Conference of Postgraduate Deans 1988) and a formal review of his progress should be carried out around two months later and at the end of the appointment.

The Joint Committee on Postgraduate Training for General Practice has now stipulated that 'Formative assessment, that is, assessment for educational purposes, should form an essential part of all posts approved or selected for general practitioner training.'

3. CLINICAL WORK

Each junior should take part in all the activities on the firm with an appropriate balance of responsibility and supervision. These activities should include the supervised assessments of emergency admissions and supervised outpatient work. Research activity is to be encouraged if it involves training in research methods and the junior staff member is to be a co-author of resulting published work.

4. EDUCATIONAL SESSIONS

Each appointee should be involved in an introductory session or induction course at the beginning of the appointment. There should also be weekly educational sessions which are separate from the routine clinical work of the firm. Consultants should be involved in these sessions and all juniors present cases and participate actively. Reading should be encouraged and journal clubs have been found to be useful. The sessions should be reviewed by District Postgraduate Medical Education Committees (Conference of Postgraduate Deans 1988).

Audits of patient care should be a regular item in the weekly educational sessions. These audits can take the form of a review of randomly chosen individual case notes but should also include a more systematic review of unit activities in such fields as prescribing, patterns of management and communications.

5. STUDY LEAVE

Study Leave should normally be made available for courses or study which is directly relevant to the agreed educational objectives . . .

6. CAREERS ADVICE AND COUNSELLING

This should be available and offered to all junior doctors in each district (Conference of Postgraduate Deans 1988).

References

Adair J. (1986). *Effective teambuilding*. Pan Books, London.

Anon (1990). A cautionary tale. *Postgraduate Education for General Practice*, (1), (2), 108–111.

Arntson, P. (1984). Preliminary findings from a study of trainer–trainee relationships in the United Kingdom.

Baillon, B. R. F., Flew, R., Hasler, J. C., Huiuis, T. J. and Toby, J. P. (1993). *Postgraduate Education for General Practice*, **4**, 29–36.

Balint, M. (1964). *The doctor, his patient and the illness*. Tavistock, London.

Belbin, R. M. (1981). *Management teams. Why they succeed or fail*. Butterworth Heinemann, Oxford.

Benner, D. (1984). *From novice to expert: excellence and power in clinical nursing practice*. Addison-Wesley, Menlo Park, California.

Berliner, D. C. (1987). Ways of thinking about students and classrooms by more and less experienced teachers. In *Exploring teachers' thinking* (ed. J. Calderhead), pp. 60–83. Cassell, London.

Berne, E. (1964). *Games people play*. Penguin Books, London.

Blanchard, K. (1990). *The one minute manager meets the monkey*. Fontana Collins, London.

Bligh, J. and Price, A. (1991). Profiling – a continuing assessment programme. *Postgraduate Education for General Practice*, **2**, 28–35.

Bloom, B. (1972). *Taxonomy of educational objectives. Handbook 1 The cognitive domain*. Longman, Harlow.

Boud, (1992). The use of self assessment schedules in negotiated learning. *Studies in Higher Education*, 17, (2).

Brown, S. and McIntyre, D. (1993). *Making sense of teaching*. Open University Press, Buckingham.

Bulstrode, C. J. K., *et al.* (1992). New deal for junior doctors' hours: how to achieve it. *British Medical Journal*, **305**, 1203–5.

Byrne, P. S. (1975). Medical and general practice. *Journal of the Royal College of General Practitioners*, **25**, 285–92.

Byrne, P. S. and Long, B. E. L. (1973). *Learning to care, person to person*. Churchill Livingstone, London.

Byrne, P. S. and Long, B. E. L. (1986). *Doctors talking to patients*. HMSO, London.

Cartwright, A. and Anderson, R. (1981). *General practice revisited*. Tavistock Publications, London.

Centre for Primary Care Research. Department of General Practice, University of Manchester (1988). *Rating Scales for Vocational Training in General Practice* RCGP Occassional Paper No. 40. RCGP, London.

Coles, C. and Holm, H. A. (1993). *Learning in medicine*. Oxford University Press, Oxford.

Conference of Postgraduate Deans (1988). *Report on Postgraduate Medical Education; a review of the educational implications of 'Achieving a balance: plan for action*.

Consumers' Association (1989). You and your GP. *Which?* **July**, 481–5.

Crawley, H. S. and Levin, J. B. (1990). Training for general practice; a national survey. *British Medical Journal*, **300**, 911–15.

Cummins, J. (1990). Learner-based self-assessment for training for general practice. *Postgraduate Education for General Practice*, **1** (2), 95–102.

Department of Health (1993). *Hospital doctors: training for the future*. The Report of the Working Group on Specialist Training. Health Publications Unit. (The Calman Report.)

Donabedian, A. (1966). Evaluating the quality of medical care. *Millbank Memorial Fund Quarterly*, **44**, 166–204.

Dreyfus, H. L. and Dreyfus, S. E. (1984). *Mind over machine*. Macmillan/The Free Press, New York.

Fabb, W. E., Herman, M. W., Phillips, W. A., and Stone, P. (1976). *Focus on learning*. Royal Australian College of General Practitioners, Melbourne.

Freeman, J. and Byrne, P. (1982). *The assessment of vocational training for general practice*. RCGP Reports from general practice 17.

Freeman, J., Roberts, J., Metcalfe, D., and Hillier, V. (1982). *The influence of trainers on trainees in general practice*. Occasional Paper RCGP, London.

Fry, J. (1979). *Common diseases*, (2nd edn). MTP Press, Lancaster.

Fuhrman B. S. and Grasha A. F. (1983). *A practical handbook for college teachers* (CHAP II 7). Boston, Mass. Little, Brown and Co.

General Medical Council (1987). *Recommendations on the training of Specialists*, GMC, London.

Godlee, F. (1992). Juniors' hours: is the end in sight? *British Medical Journal*, **305**, 937–40.

Grant, J., Marsden, P., and King P. C. (1989). Senior house officers and their training *British Medical Journal*, **289**, 1265–8.

Guillebaud. (1985) *Contraception: your questions answered*. Churchill-Livingstone, Edinburgh.

Hall, M. S. (ed.) (1983). *A. G. P. training handbook* Ch. 16, p. 111. Blackwell Scientific Publications, Oxford.

Harris, T. A. (1970). *I'm OK, You're OK*. Pan Books, London.

Hart, J. T. (1988). *A new kind of doctor*. Merlin Press, London.

Hasler, J. C. (1983). Do trainees see patients with chronic illness? *British Medical Journal*, **287**, 1679–82.

Hasler, J. C. (1989). The history of vocational training for general practice: the seventies and eighties. *Journal of the Royal College of General Practitioners*, **39**, 338–41.

Hitchcock, G. (1988). *Profiles and profiling: a practice introduction*. Longman, Harlow.

Hodgkin, K. (1985). *Towards earlier diagnosis*, (5th edn). Churchill Livingstone, Edinburgh.

Honey, P. and Mumford, A. (1986). *Using your learning styles*, (2nd edn). Peter Honey, Maidenhead.

Horder, J. P. and Swift, G. (1979). The history of vocational training for general practice. *Journal of the Royal College of General Practitioners*, **29**, 24–32.

Kearly, K. (1990). An evaluation of the hospital component of general practice vocational training. *British Journal of General Practice*, **40**, 409–14.

Kolb, D. *et al.* (1974). *Organisational psychology: an experiential approach*. Prentice Hall, London.

Lipsy R. (1988). *An art of our own: the spiritual in twentieth century art*. Shambula Publications, Boston, Mass.

McCormick, J. (1979). *The doctor, father figure or plumber*. Croom Helm, London.

McWhinney, I. R. (1966). General practice as an academic discipline. *The Lancet*, **1**, 419–23.

Mann, K. J. (1966). The role of the family and community health centre. *Bulletin New York Academy of Medicine*, **42**, (2), 742.

Marinker M. (1981). Vocational trainees. In *Teaching general practice*, (ed. J. Cormack, M. Marinker, and D. Morrell). Kluwer Medical, London.

Metcalfe, D. H. H. (1989). The Edinburgh declaration. *Family Practice*, **6**(3), 165–6.

Mezirow, J. (1981). A critical theory of adult learning and education. *Adult Education*, **32**, 3–24.

Morrell, D. C. (1989). Sir David Bruce Memorial Lecture. *Journal of the Royal Army Medical Corps*, **135**, 43.

Morrell, D. (1988). *Epidemiology in general practice*. Oxford University Press.

Munro K. (1992). *Teamworking in practice*. Radcliffe Medical Press, Oxford.

National Health Service Management Executive (1991). *Working for patients: postgraduate and continuing medical and dental education*. Health Publications Unit, Heywood, Lancashire.

Neighbour, R. (1987). *The inner consultation*. MTP Press, Lancaster.

Nolan, V. (1987). *Teamwork*. Sphere Reference Books, London.

O' Dowd, T. C. and Wilson, A. D. (1991). Set menus and clinical freedom. *British Medical Journal*, **303**, 450–2.

Oxford Region Course Organisers and Advisers Group (1988). *Priority objectives for vocational training*, (2nd edn). RCGP Occasional Paper No. 30. RCGP, London.

Patterson, L. J. and Hajela, V. P. (1992). Formal appraisal of junior medical staff. *Journal of the Royal College of Physicians of London*, **26**, (4), 383–4.

Pendleton, D. A., Schofield, T. P. C., Tate, P. H. C., and Havelock, P. B. (1984). *The consultation. An approach to learning and teaching*. Oxford University Press GP Series 6. OUP, Oxford.

Pereira Gray, D. J. (1979). *A system of training for general practice*, (2nd edn). RCGP Occasional Paper No. 4 RCGP, London.

Pereira Gray, O. (1982). *Training for general practice*. Chapter 20. McDonald and Evans, Plymouth.

Pritchard, P. Low, K., and Whalen, M. (1984). *Management in general practice*. Oxford University Press, GP Series 8. OUP, Oxford.

Rashid, A., *et al.* (1989). Consultations in general practice: a comparison of patients' and doctors' satisfaction. *British Medical Journal*, **299**, 1015–16.

RCGP (1972). *The future general practitioner*. BMA, London.

RCGP (1981). *Health and prevention in Primary Care*. Report from General Practice No. 18. RCGP, London.

RCGP (1985). *What sort of doctor?* RCGP occasional paper 23.

RCGP (1981 and 1982). Occasional Papers 18–22, RCGP, London.

RCGP (1993). Series of booklets on the Hospital component of vocational training. RCGP, London.

Reeve, H. and Bowman, A. (1989). Hospital training for general practice: views of trainees in the North Western Region. *British Medical Journal*, **298**, 1432–4.

Ronalds, C., Douglas, A., Gray, D. P. and Shelley, P. Fourth National Trainee Conference. Occasional Paper 18. London: Royal College of General Practitioners, 1981.

Royal Commission on Medical Education (1968). Report. HMSO, London.

Samuel, O. (1990). *Towards a curriculum for general practice training*. RCGP Occasional Paper No. 44. RCGP, London.

Schein, E. (1973). *Professional education*. McGraw Hill, New York

Schofield, T. P. C. and Hasler, J. C. (1984). Approval of trainers and training practices in the Oxford Region. *British Medical Journal*, **288**, 538–40. 614–8. 688–9.

Schon, D. A. (1983). *The reflective practitioner*. Basic Books, New York.
SCOPME (1991). *Improving the experience – good practice in SHO training*. SCOPME, London.
SCOPME (1992). *Formal opportunities in postgraduate education for hospital doctors in training*. SCOPME, London.
Second European Conference on the Teaching of General Practice (1974). *The general practitioner in Europe*. Leeuwenhorst, The Netherlands.
Skeff, K. M., Berman, J., and Stratos, R. (1988). A review of clinical teaching improvement methods and a theoretical framework for their evaluation. In *Clinical teaching for medical residents: roles, techniques and programs*, (ed. J. C. Edwards and R. L. Marier). Springer, New York.
Styles, W. M. (1988). *Vocational training for general practice – hospital experience*. A report from the Joint Committee on Postgraduate Training for General Practice. JCPTGP, London.
Sutherland, V. T. and Cooper, C. L. (1992). Job stress, satisfaction and mental health among general practitioners before and after the introduction of the new contract. *British Medical Journal*, **304**, 1545–8.
Tate, P. H. L. and Pendleton, D. A. (1980). Why not tear up the European Aims? *Journal of the Royal College of General Practitioners*, **30**, 743.
Tibbot, C., Smith, P., and Robert, G. (1990). The mutually agreed support system (MARS). *Postgraduate Education for General Practice*, **1**, 42–5.
Tom, A. (1984). *Teaching as a moral craft*. Longman, New York.
Tudor Hart, J. (1988). *A new kind of doctor*. Merlin Press, London.
Turnberg, L. A. (1992). Education and training for Senior House Officers. *Journal of the Royal College of Physicians of London*, **26**, (2), 188–91.
Weed, L. L. (1969). *Medical records, medical education and patient care*. Press of Case Western Reserve University, Cleveland.
Zander L. I., Beresford, S. A. A., and Thomas, P. (1978). *Medical records in general practice*. RCGP Occasional Paper No. 5. RCGP. London.
Zeichner, K. M., Tabachnick, R. M., and Densmore, K. (1987). Individual, institutional and cultural influences on the development of teachers craft knowledge. In *Exploring teachers' thinking* (ed. J. Calderhead), pp. 21–59. Cassell, London.

Index